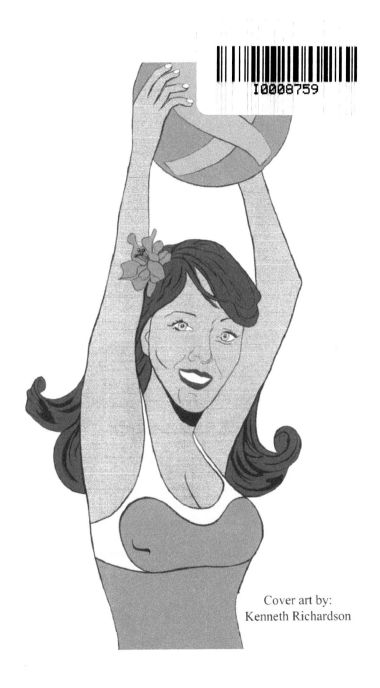

I0008759

Cover art by:
Kenneth Richardson

LIVE AND GIVE:

Facebooking My Way Through Breast Cancer

HOLLY ROSE

Dedication

There are so many people who helped me along the way; Shelley and her Facebook posting, my girls who kept me laughing and living, Katie, Julie, Gretchen, Leslie and Janeen, who listened to me endlessly, my Doctors, who worked their magic, especially Dr. Zannis, who treated me with care and kindness, and everyone on Facebook with their warm wishes and prayers who kept my spirits up everyday. They all deserve thanks, but the one person I have to dedicate this to is my dear, sweet, hubby John. He has been my source of strength through every moment. I admire him so for his strength, I respect him as a father, I love him as husband, and I adore him as a man. I'm the luckiest girl in the world to have him.

Introduction

I never once fancied myself a writer, but something happened to me during my experience with breast cancer. After my first surgery I began writing to fight off depression and, to my amazement, the words poured out of me. I wrote every thought, every moment, every emotion I felt: happy, sad, scared, angry, tired and triumphant. In seventeen days I had a book in my hand.

I spent the rest of the year editing it with the help of my dear friend Katie. During the course of the year, I discovered I had a passion for writing and couldn't help but continue to write. While waiting for replies from editors, I began working on my sequel to "Live and Give", continuing to chronicle my journey through chemotherapy and radiation.

After receiving a few very kind and encouraging rejections, I decided to give it a go on my own and to self-publish "Live and Give." I didn't have the patience to wait to snag an editor, who would then tell me to wait while they snagged a publisher, who would tell me to wait for my turn in their timeline. After what I have been through, I don't take a day for granted.

Once I decided to self-publish, I chose to combine the two books. My decision was, again, partly based on the realization that I have no guarantee on the number of days I have in this lifetime (no one does).

Part One and Part Two were written at completely different times in my journey and carry distinct undercurrents of each time period. I was inspired to write Part One, and the words came out with ease writing over hundred pages in seventeen days. Part Two, on the other hand, was very difficult for me to write. I cried recalling each event, and I cried more while editing it, and I'm sure I'll cry reading it in the future. The two parts together represent my entire experience with breast cancer and my journey through this wonderful life.

I can't explain it, but I believe God decided to give me a voice. He gave me something to say at that moment in time and I felt compelled to write it down. Maybe it's my story that will save one more mother, one more wife, one more daughter, one more sister, one more friend, one more woman . . . one more life.

It's ironic that I'm thankful for this whole experience. I am grateful for my lessons learned and I am thankful to share my journey with you. My hope is that you enjoy reading it and walk away from this book with an appreciation for your life, every day of it. And, of course, I want you to: "Don't be a Chump! Check for a Lump!"

Part I
Live and Give

Chapter One

"Why me? Why me?" That is what I kept asking myself. "Why me?"

At the beginning of this I wanted to keep a journal every day to write down every experience, good and bad. If I had to go through this, Damn it! I was going to get something out of it. Every day I said, "I will write tonight," and every night I had so many emotions thrashing about that it was impossible for me to start. It was impossible to do anything until it was out. (It is still hard for me to say the word. I am hoping I am cancer free now. I just had my surgery three days ago. I'm still asking "Why me?") Now, I hope I can recall all of my emotions and details clearly and in sequence.

Tuesday, January 13th, 2009. I sat at my computer that afternoon procrastinating on Facebook. In case you are one of the few, who have not discovered Facebook yet, it is a website that helps you connect and share with people in your life on the Internet. On the site, users are able to compile a list of their friends, both old and new. Each person's personal postings, comments, and photo albums allow you to see and interact within your own friend network. My girlfriend Shelley, a good friend since the 6th grade, posted on Facebook a picture that would forever change my life. On January 13th, 2009 at 1:36 p.m Shelley posted a playful posting from a breast cancer awareness non-profit reminding me to perform a self-breast check.

Everyone on Facebook made funny comments about Shelley's posting, my husband, John Rose, included.

Joe Sounds good to me!

Tricia Who's gonna watch me feel my boobs?

John Rose Do man-boobs count?

Shelley invited us all to join the group on Facebook, which I did. It may have saved my life.

That next night I recalled the posting and I did feel my boobies. To my horror, I found a lump. I asked my husband John to feel it, thinking he touches my boobs more than I do, and he'll know if it's a lump. He said he didn't notice anything different. Keeping up on my self-checks had always been a chore for me. I probably did a self-check three - four times a year. My breasts were so lumpy to begin with that I never thought I would be able to feel anything anyway. This sure did feel like something though. I went to sleep with the lump looming in the back of my mind.

The next morning I woke up and the first thing I did was feel for the lump again. I knew this was NOT nothing. It felt like one of those hard bouncy balls, the kind you buy for a quarter from a gumball machine, was inside my left breast. Immediately I called my gynecologist. The receptionist asked me why I was making an appointment. I told her I had found a lump.

Then she asked, "How big is the lump? The size of a pea, a dime, a nickel?" "Oh crap!" I had to tell them it was much larger. My mind started racing at that point. It was so much larger than a pea. What the hell? Fear started to creep up on me. The receptionist quickly said she would get me in that day. She took my home and cell phone numbers and said she would call back that day with an appointment time.

"Crap!! I have a lump in my breast! Crap! I have a lump in my breast. This isn't happening!"

I waited by the phone all day long. Twelve o'clock passed, it was still early. 1:00 . . . 2:00. "It can't possibly be cancer. It must be a cyst or something." I didn't want to be rude and call again. They knew the importance. I was going to let them do their job. 3:00 . . . 4:00. "What is taking so long?" Now I was anxious and needed to get out of the house. Our girls, Hannah (11) and Ivy (10), had tennis at 4:30, so my hubby suggested we drop off the kids at tennis and go to the club and have a drink to mellow out. I had given my cell phone number to the receptionist and my husband's cell phone number as well, so I figured, "What the hell, a drink would do me good."

John and I went to the club and relaxed. We sat outside looking over the golf course as we usually did and commented on how good life was. John and I often stopped and realized how good we had it, how lucky we were, in everything; our life, our kids, each other, our house, our free time . . . you name it, we felt fortunate. We held hands a little tighter that day. I tried to keep a smile on and not think about it. My strong hubby gave me confidence that I was going to be okay. "It just can't be cancer. It just can't be. I'm too positive of a person to get cancer. That would blow my whole theory that happy people don't get cancer. Granted, I had never known any adults personally that had cancer, so my theory wasn't very credible."

The call never came. We gathered up our kids and went back home. I assumed at this point, that I didn't have much time left to get into the office, so I called back. Their answering machine picked up with a message that they were closed and to call back during regular hours. I then checked my messages and sure enough they had called the minute we left for tennis. Why they didn't call my cell phone or my husband's cell phone is beyond me. "HELLO? I found a lump in my breast. Can you not dial one other number? This was no pea-sized lump, it was a bouncy ball!!!"

I had talked to a few friends throughout the day and everyone told me the same statistic that eighty percent of all lumps are nothing, just cysts or benign lumps. No big deal. Each person recounted that they knew two or three people who found lumps and each time it was nothing. My friends and I were at the age for health problems to begin arising.

Twenty days earlier, I had turned thirty-nine years old. My birthday was the day after Christmas, December 26th. Growing up having a Christmas birthday I had always felt jipped, receiving the famous Christmas/birthday combo presents. All of my birthday presents were even wrapped in Christmas wrapping paper – no pink, no polka dots, no paisley. No one wanted to celebrate anything, including my birthday, once Christmas was finally over. Birthdays were supposed to be special-even it was on the day after Christmas.

Every year I had these awesome expectations that John would surprise me with special gifts, exciting events for the day and a fabulous cake. Year after year I was disappointed. Not that John didn't shower me with presents or attention to celebrate my birthday, because he did treat me wonderful every year. I think I was just expecting something spectacular each year to make up for my bummer birthdays, having it the day after Christmas. I wanted my birthday to be special.

This year it was special. In fact, it was the best birthday I'd ever had! To ensure my birthday was exactly what I wanted it to be, I took charge and planned every moment of my day. It was perfect and I must add that John and the girls made it all perfect. They catered to my every whim. My lazy morning was spent doing a puzzle with Hannah and Ivy. (Yes, I love puzzles. I admit it. Santa brings me a puzzle every year.) Later, John and our girls and I went out to dinner to a local Greek restaurant. Music filled the air as the band played. We joyously shared stories and laughter. My smile could not have been any bigger when John rose from the table and the next thing I knew he had the microphone in hand. My sweet hubby was serenading me with the loveliest rendition of Happy Birthday I had ever heard. I didn't care that I was getting older. I didn't care that I had wrinkles or grey hair or an extra twenty pounds. I had everything I ever wanted out of life right in front of me - John, Hannah and Ivy.

I would have been perfectly satisfied ending the night right then and there, and I would have recalled it as the best birthday in my thirty-nine years. Although, that was not the end of the night, it had just begun. We dropped the girls off at home with a babysitter and John and I went to the bowling alley with some good friends. The balls kept a rollin' and the drinks kept a comin' that night. We laughed harder and harder as the night went on. Every twenty minutes or so I would tell one of my girlfriends, "Did I tell you my hubby sang to me?" I loved him so. He made me feel extra special this birthday. It truly was the best Birthday ever!!!!

Here I was three weeks later worried that I might have cancer. I hung on to the thought that eighty percent are nothing, and I survived the day and night.

That evening I told John it was time to call his mom, Carol. She is an angelic woman with a very kind and giving spirit. I wasn't sure I wanted to tell everyone just yet, but I was getting a little scared. John called his mom and requested that she start the prayer chain moving. If anyone could rally up many prayers fast it was Carol. And she sure did.

The next morning, first thing when I woke up, I again felt the lump. This was definitely something. Worry was sinking in deeper. I had spa day planned for that morning with the "sisters de Rosa" (The Rose sisters, or Rose wives I should say). John's family consists of six boys, one girl (who is the oldest), his mother Carol, who is married to Glenn and living in Salt Lake City, Utah, and his father Marv, who is married to Margarita and living here in Phoenix. So, when we had a girl's day out we usually had four or five women show up. We often commented on how lucky we were, to be able to have that many wives get together and all get along. Today was our annual spa day with all of the Rose women attending (except for John's mom who was in Utah).

I wasn't quite up for spa day. I needed to get into the doctor's office first and find out what this was, before I could relax. I called John's sister, Brenda, to break the news that I wasn't going to attend. She is the one we all call. She instantaneously takes care of business. She always understands. She is always there if you need her. If you are stuck on an island and can choose only one person to help you get off, she is the person you want to choose. She lives by the credo, "just do what is right" there is no other option. It's not even an option to think about another option. I think that applies to everything in her life, her family, her kids, her marriage, her religion, her friends, her house . . . everything. I respect and admire her for it. Living admirably is not an easy task and she does it showing very little effort. I just love her and her husband, Brandon.

I phoned Brenda first thing in the morning telling her I didn't think I could make it to spa day. After I explained why, she had encouraging words for me. She told me not to worry, that she would explain it to everyone and that she would be saying prayers for me. I said I would try to make it late to spa day if I was able to get into the doctor's office early and received good news. I told her I would call later.

I hung up with Brenda and called my ob/gyn next. I spoke with someone new and told my story again about how I had waited all day the day before. She booked me right away, telling me to get there as soon as I could. Quickly, I got myself ready. I stood before my hubby, with my toes pointed inward as I did when I was uneasy, shaking my hands up and down nervously saying, "Eighty percent are nothing. Eighty percent are nothing, right?" He told me everything would be fine. I hugged my hubby and off I went. I kept repeating, "Eighty percent are nothing. Eighty percent are nothing" all the way there. "Crap! Eighty percent are nothing. Crap!" Fifteen minutes later I arrived at the office.

While checking myself in, I had to explain again to the receptionist what my appointment was for and why I was not on the books. I sat down in the waiting room mindlessly flipping through a magazine, but my attention was elsewhere. Questions started popping up in my head. "I wonder if the people in the waiting area just heard that? I wonder what they are thinking. Are they looking at me like I have cancer? Oh my gosh!!! I could have cancer. Eighty percent are nothing. Eighty percent are nothing! Just one! Just one!"

Just one! is a phrase I repeat to myself when I feel like I'm going to cry in public. It came from a story my girlfriend told me years ago. I'll tell it to you now, even though you probably won't find it funny or give a damn, but maybe you can find your "Just one" phrase to help you get through your life.

Here goes: My friend's younger sister loved food. Not just sweets mind you; she liked steak and fried chicken. To help explain just how much she liked food she told me how her mother had warned her sister of Stranger Danger. He tempted little kids to get into his car and then take them far, far away. She warned Stranger Danger would entice little kids with ice cream, with candy AND with chicken. Not sure about you, but I don't think I would have stepped into a stranger's car because he had a roasted chicken in hand. Apparently, her little sister would have climbed into a stranger's car for chicken. This was how much she liked her food. One evening when at KFC, her mother ordered food to go. The daughter couldn't wait to get home to eat, so she asked her mother if she could have a leg for the road. Her mother said "No."

The daughter repeated again and again in a childlike slur/lisp, "Just one! Just one! Just a leg! Just a leg! Just one!" I still laugh when I think of this story. It has remained with me for years.

I repeat "Just one!" anytime I don't want to embarrass myself by crying in public.

Advice #1: Find your "Just one".

My usual doctor, who I love, was not there that day so I

had to see another doctor. She was equally nice and made me feel very comfortable. She did the breast exam on my right breast first, talking to me the whole time, then the left breast.

She immediately found the lump and calmly told me, "Oh, this feels like a cyst. This totally feels like a cyst. You have nothing to worry about." Looking back, if she did have a clue that it was cancer I was very thankful that she didn't lead on. The next couple of nights were the last few nights of restful sleep I had without the help of some kind of anxiety or sleeping medicine to get me through the night. She didn't allow me to leave until I had peace of mind that the lump was nothing to worry about. She had me feel it, and then had me feel my right side, showing me how they were similar somehow and how it moved. I wasn't sure I agreed with her, but she did quell my worries. She had me do some other blood work and my normal pap, and then advised me that I needed to go to the specialist to do a mammogram "just to make sure". Her office didn't do digital mammograms there, so I had to go somewhere else. I left the doctor's office feeling good. They say ignorance is bliss, and it was for a few days.

As soon as I walked out of the office, I called John with the good news. He said, "I knew it!" I still wasn't up for spa day. I felt like I had been on an emotional roller coaster. I needed a moment alone, to let all of my emotions settle. Brenda was my next call. That morning, I was crying to her because I thought I might have cancer. Then later that day, I was crying to her because I was going to live. She told me she had been crying too on the way to spa day. She was already planning on how she could help John raise the girls, etc.- just in case.

I immediately made my appointment for my mammogram for the 22nd of January. That was almost a week away. I spent the week not worrying. Everyone had asked how it went at my doctor's appointment and I responded each time with "Good news! The doctor says it looks like a cyst, but to check it out, just to make sure." No problem. No worries. The week went on. Life as usual - school, tennis lessons, workouts, dinners, birthday parties, facebooking, etc.

That Sunday, we had dinner with a few of our neighbors, Chip and Janeen (and their three sons) and Todd and Leslie (and their son and daughter). We couldn't have moved in next to better people three years ago. Our evening together was fabulous. We had lots of food, lots of wine, and lots of fun. By the end of the evening I told the gals about my scare finding a lump and how it was nothing. Janeen, and her usual bold self, asked to feel it. I thought she was kidding. And she said, "No, I want to know what it feels like in case I ever feel anything." I consented and let her and Leslie feel my lump. They both told me how they never did breast exams because they felt they had lumpy breasts to begin with and didn't think they would ever be able to tell a difference anyway. I informed them that was exactly what I used to think. Let me tell you, you will know the difference. In the past month I have had woman after woman tell me the exact same thing, time and time again. Don't fool yourselves girls. You will know your body and for us lumpy gals there's even more reason to do self-checks.

Advice #2: Don't be a Chump! Check for a Lump!

Chapter Two

Saturday, January 19th, 2009. Today was my daughter Ivy's 10th birthday. We had a surprise party for her at the amusement park with her friends over the weekend. My belief is that your official birthday only comes once a year, and must be commemorated, even if you did have a party on another day. So, to celebrate Ivy's official birthday I took her and Hannah to the mall. Ivy had her ears pierced that afternoon, which was her birthday present. As the clerk stood in front of her with the piercing gun, I watched her innocent little face shrivel up with fear. In one quick second it was over and Ivy was admiring her new sparkly ears in a mirror.

Ivy had always been our little fashionista, enjoying the glitz and the glam. Early on she would piece together crazy ensembles that only she could pull off. Donned in her tights and her knee-high boots and her flowered prints she would casually throw her glittery scarf around her neck, flipping her hair around as she did so and in her deep throaty voice pronounce, "I'm ready mom."

I relished every moment that day watching them. Not a minute with them was going to pass me by. I soaked up their twinkling tween spirit like a sponge. As they giggled and shared stories from school with me I thought, "I may not be here one day to do this. I may not be here to listen to them talk about boys or the drama with their friends. Who will be there to give them advice and help steer them through the rough waters? WHO?" I panicked. "I needed to teach them everything - quickly!" Throughout the day I kept inserting little messages into our conversation about boys, friendships, integrity and life in general. One more lesson I could get in, just in case. I love them both so much. They really are my life and my reason for living.

I'll never forget the exact moment I decided to have

children. John and I were living in Las Vegas at the time. I was driving home on the freeway from my shift at the casino as a cigarette girl, when on my right I came upon a car wreck. This was not just a fender bender mind you, but a massive crumpled pile of metal. The driver's side was beyond recognition. Horrified, I thought the person driving the car must be dead. In one instant their life gone, just like that, and then I had a selfish thought. What if that car had been me, or worse yet, what if that car had been John's? What if John was in a terrible car wreck and died? How I would miss him so. I couldn't bare living without him. As I stared at the wreck before me, I thought about the dreadful idea of living without him and I realized, then and there, I had to have his baby. Not just wanted to, but HAD to. I ached to have part of him to live on in case something tragic ever occurred. I couldn't imagine going on without him - alone. I wanted HIS baby.

John was the love of my life. There were other boyfriends before him but no one that I allowed myself to love. No one that I had ever felt like I could let my wall down enough and let them love me. John made me feel safe and secure like no one else ever had. I didn't have to put on any pretenses with him. He gave me unconditional approval in every way. I could be me.

He made such an astounding impression on me on our first date. On the drive over to his house butterflies filled my stomach. Many hours of contemplation and consultation with friends had been spent deciding the perfect outfit. The winning ensemble was a black bodysuit with a scalloped v-neck in the front and the back, worn with my favorite Gap jeans and some black boots (remember this was 1992). I stepped out of the car, flipped my bright red hair over, fluffing up my long spiral perm, and excitedly walked to the door. He opened the door looking just as cute as could be in his vintage Levi striped shorts and tank t-shirt. His tank exposed his Warhol/Velvet Underground banana tattoo on his shoulder. I had never been much for tattoos on men, but this was a banana – it made me laugh. He stood there with a smile and a single red rose for me.

I thanked him and he responded with "Yah, well." We then jumped into my car to go see a band (Major Lingo). Once in the car he asked if he could pop in a cassette (again, remember this was 1992). Most men would have popped in the latest and greatest trying to impress me, but not John. A moment later out poured John Travolta and Olivia Newton John. He played the Grease soundtrack. Right then and there, I knew this was a man I wanted to get to know better. He was a little on the wild side, yet wholesome and pure at the same time. He was confident, secure, incredibly funny, super charming, handsome as could be, and just cool as all hell. Two weeks later he moved in with me and the rest is history.

Here we were seventeen years later, January 21st, about to celebrate our thirteenth Anniversary together. It was the night before my next doctor's appointment. Being a little (okay very) superstitious, I think I may have jinxed myself. I had posted on Facebook:

> Holly Toner-Rose 13 can be a lucky
> number too.

I tempted luck. Not sure why I did this. I wonder if things would have been different had I not posted that. Silly superstitions. Fearing bad luck would find me, twenty minutes later I changed my post to:

> Holly Toner-Rose I'm a True Believer!

I was a true believer in John and our love. Along with my posting I included the link to a Half Japanese song; the sweet song that was playing when John proposed to me. It was deep in the night while we were driving to Utah. We were both silent as we listened to the romantic tunes pour out of the stereo. Out of nowhere John picked up my hand, and while stroking it he asked, "If I asked you to marry me would you?"

Shocked and excited by what I thought might be ahead, I replied smiling with "Is this a proposal?"

"What if it was? Would you say yes?"

"I don't know. You'd have to ask me first."

With the loving melody playing in the background, he said the four little words that I had been waiting for "Will you marry me?"

I happily burst out "YES!" Happy tears came to my eyes as he kissed me. I'll never forget that he thanked me for saying yes. I don't know if he thought there was a chance I was going to say no. Silly boy, of course, I would say yes.

We stopped at the next gas station and John yelled out to the gas station attendant, "She's gonna marry me! I just asked her to marry me and she said yes!" Not having planned out his proposal he didn't have a ring on hand, so he stopped at the gumball machine and bought me a twenty-five cent ring. I was as happy as could be.

A few months later John and I made our plans to elope. We made our way up the coast of California. On January 21st, 1996 we were married in a chapel, an old rustic barn, in Harmony, California. Population seventeen. It was the happiest day of my life. I was Mrs. John Marvin Rose. I was his wife and he was my husband. We were married!

Fourteen years had passed since that very special day and I would say yes all over again. That night, we made love, and I forgot about the lump and luck and everything else. I was still madly in love with my hubby.

Thursday, January 22nd, 2009, the day of my mammogram appointment. Thoughts sped through my mind that morning. "Maybe I should be scared and maybe I didn't give this enough attention. Maybe I was supposed to realize something those first few days and have already made a change in my life. Was God mad that I didn't make a change or see what it was that I was supposed to see in all of this? Crap! I should have been worried this whole week and have done something different to ensure today would be good. Maybe I should have changed. Maybe I should have spent more time with my kids or spent more time with John. What was I thinking? Why was I taking life for granted this whole week? I didn't change a thing! Wait. Eighty percent are nothing."

My appointment was late in the afternoon. I told John he didn't need to go with me. First he was offended and then I explained that I would just wind up crying if he went, being the emotional, sappy person I am. It was going to be nothing anyway. My friend Katie and sister-in-law Carol offered to go with me too. Again, I declined. Off I went.

I checked in for my appointment. Today I was getting a digital mammogram and an ultrasound. I was expecting good news and for this all to be over within an hour or two. First, I had my mammogram. A mammogram is an x-ray image taken of your breast in order to visualize normal and abnormal structures, including cancer. In order to take the x-ray image, a patient's breast is placed in between two flat panels and then the panels are compressed until your boob is one big pancake. (Ouch!)

The woman who performed the mammogram was very pleasant. We talked about kids, etc, the whole time. I still had no worries. Nothing hurt, I felt good. I was in the best shape of my life. After she was done she directed me to the waiting room, still in my gown, to wait for the ultrasound. I had brought a book with me so I was patiently reading - not worrying. About fifteen minutes later the woman who gave me the mammogram walked past me and gently squeezed my shoulder and told me it wasn't going to be too much longer in a soft soothing tone. "Something was wrong with her squeeze. She squeezed a little too hard. Why didn't I bring John with me? Why did she squeeze my shoulder so empathetically? And what was with her soft tone? Crap! She saw something bad." (My heart is beating faster reliving this.) "Where is John? Maybe I should call him. Why was I so stupid not to bring him with me? Just one! Just one! She squeezed too hard. Okay Holly, calm down. Eighty percent are nothing. It's going to be fine. Just one!"

The next technician called me in. He informed me he

would be doing my ultrasound that day. An ultrasound produces pictures of the inside of the body through high frequency sound waves. I watched the screen intently the entire time trying to make out what I saw. I had seen ultrasounds done before on me, when I was pregnant with my kids and once for a heart check. I knew that I was not able to read them, but I sure did try. I noticed something that looked like tissue and then a black mark. "Can a black mark be good? Is that what a cyst looks like? A cyst is a build up of some type of fluid or tissue. It could look black, right? It's not a water cyst like someone suggested. Water wouldn't be black. Just one! It will be fine," I reassured myself. The doctor took a few pictures and measurements. He told me to stay there, that he was going to check with the doctor to see if he wanted anything else before I changed back into my clothes.

At this point, while lying on the bed with a paper garment draped over my chest, I repeated "Just one. Just one. Just one. Why didn't I bring John? Please God! Just one! Just one! Why was I so stupid not to bring John? Just . . . ". In walked the ultrasound technician with the doctor in tow. Right then I knew "Holy Crap! I have cancer! This doctor didn't need to come in here unless something was wrong. I NEED JOHN!!!!"

The doctor made no hesitation and very coldly said to me, "What I see is not very good. Prepare yourself for a long hard road. All I can tell you is to be strong."

My mind sped frantically. "He is telling me I have cancer. What??????? He is telling me I have cancer. Oh God! I need John!!! Where is John? I have cancer!"

Then he said "I don't sugar coat anything for my patients. I tell it like I see it. You have a long hard road ahead of you. Silver lining is you have large breasts so they should be able to save your breast. Do you have any questions? I can sit here as long as you like to answer questions."

"Was he kidding? Did I have questions?" I only had two thoughts rolling through my mind. "Crap! I have Cancer!"

21

and "Where is John? I need John!" and a third thought, "Asshole!" Beyond that, my mind was frozen. His voice was void of any emotion whatsoever. "How can he sit here and tell me I have cancer in his icy voice."

A few seconds later I responded that I didn't have any questions. My mind was so shaken, that I couldn't produce a coherent question had I tried. He informed me that I needed to have a biopsy done, but unfortunately they didn't have the equipment there. I was told his office would call my ob/gyn to set up the appointment and someone would call me first thing in the morning. He said hopefully they could squeeze me in the next day (Friday) or Monday if not. I was then instructed that I could change back into my clothes and the ultrasound tech would show me out.

Left alone in the room I tried to stay composed knowing I had to pass through the lobby. "I have cancer!!! I need John!!!!! I need John!!!!!!" Quickly, I put my pretty purple shirt on, not feeling so pretty anymore. My body was shaking. Fear was running through every vein inside me. I took a deep breath, pushing back the tears, said "Just one." and reached for the doorknob. Once I opened the door I saw the ultrasound tech there to my left, who, when I reached him, just pointed the way to the lobby. "Gee thanks!" is all I have to say to that. Briskly, I walked passed the lobby full of patients, hoping I could make it out of the door before the tears started to flow. I made it out with a quiver. My body was trembling when I reached the car and I began to sob. "I have cancer." With my phone already in hand I called John. When he answered I was completely speechless, I just cried and cried.

John asked "What happened honey?"

I stuttered, "I-I-I have cancer."

I think he replied with, "Oooh honey." He calmed me as best he could on the phone. He wanted to know where I was. I didn't know. Everything around me was a complete blur; buildings, cars and people were passing me by in a haze. A doctor just told me I had cancer!!! I asked John to find a place for the kids to go. Our children didn't need to witness mommy in hysterics. No sense in scaring them, yet. We both said, "I love you" and hung up.

Driving home I sobbed hysterically. More sobbing and more sobbing. I thought to myself I must look ridiculous to all of these rush hour drivers. I didn't care. "They just told me I have cancer!!!!!!!!!!!!!!!!!!!!!!!!! I don't want to die!!!!!!! The sobbing never stopped. I was hardly able to drive since I couldn't see much with the tears pouring out of me. Compounded with my hysteria, I was a virtual driving hazard. It's amazing I made it home that day in my reckless state, which is one more reason to bring someone with you to these appointments.

John called me back to let me know that the girls were going to stay the night at Uncle Stephen and Aunt Alisha's. I needed John. I had always thought of myself as being strong and independent, but that was just a mask. John is really my strength. I needed him. I raced to reach him, knowing he would make it all better, he always did. I was almost home now.

Advice #3:   Bring someone with you to any doctor's appointments that have ANY possibility of receiving bad results.

Still sobbing, I pulled up to my driveway. I walked in the door and John looked at me lovingly. Instantly, I fell into his arms. He gently cradled my left breast in his hand. I almost felt that his love could heal me and make it all better. I sobbed in his arms for an eternity. His strong embrace reassured me I would be okay.

Neither one of us wanted to cook, so, we jumped in the car to go out to eat somewhere. We kept driving from place to place. No place seemed to be perfect. I didn't want a big crowd in case I started to cry in public. I didn't want to be far from home since I felt like drinking my troubles away and I think my hubby did too. Yet, I didn't want to be any place that we would see people we knew, since I knew tears were sure to come out at some point. We ended up at the club again. It was our peaceful place. We would sit on the patio overlooking the pond and the vast array of greenery around us. It was beautiful. We held hands tighter than before and looked at each other lovingly. He told me everything would be fine. I would be fine. I said "Okay." and held his hand tighter and tighter.

John asked me all the questions: what they did, what they said, etc., etc. I realized I didn't even know where I had gone. The name of the office was a total blank to me. It all happened in a flash. The office I visited didn't leave me with one scrap of paper. No phone number, no hotline, no office number - diddley squat! I'm still a little bitter about that. "If you are going to tell someone they have cancer, and tell them rudely at that, the least they can do is offer a piece of paper with a phone number. That way, by chance I have questions, once I have processed a minute amount of this, I would have a number to call in hand. Of course, I had questions now! My husband had questions! Why didn't they give me one $%^*@$!* number?" My handsome hubby comforted me some more. He then took charge and became my medical advocate. I'm so proud and thankful for having him by my side.

By the next morning John had made calls to my ob/gyn, found out where I had gone, called his uncle who worked for the Mayo Clinic to get his advice, called his mother to start the prayer chain going again, and who knows who else. We figured out at some point that the doctor never did indeed say that I had cancer. He was just speculating. There was still a chance that it was benign. A doctor had to do a biopsy to confirm anything. A biopsy entailed removing a piece of my breast tissue that was questionable for cancer. The doctors would send this tissue to a lab and perform the necessary tests to validate if it was indeed cancer, and if so, the type of cancer. John's uncle, who is a radiologist, also confirmed this and said that eighty percent of biopsies come back nothing. That is a large percentage. Why did that doctor say, "You have a long hard road ahead of you?" His words kept ringing in my head. I went back and forth the next few days, confident I didn't have cancer and confident I did.

We anxiously waited for a call that morning from my ob/gyn to give us the details of my next appointment. After John had made several calls, he realized that no one was processing my chart. Apparently, someone was waiting for insurance approval to make the appointment. John found out after many calls later, that we didn't need approval through our insurance. He spoke with a supervisor back and forth, back and forth, and he was finally able to make the appointment. They first told my husband that the next available appointment was two and a half weeks away. He told them they were crazy and that we were willing to go anywhere to get in quicker. He very firmly said "No way are we waiting that long!" He fought with them and for me and booked me an appointment for Wednesday the 28th. Today was Friday the 23rd - five more days. Again, I'm not sure what I would have done without him. Actually I do, I would have waited two and a half weeks for my next appointment. When you think you may have cancer and are waiting for results, let me tell you, every day is a lifetime.

Advice #4: Fight for sooner appointments. Better yet, have someone else fight for you. You need a medical advocate during this difficult time.

Chapter Three

Five torturous days were ahead of me. I tried to fill my days, to prevent myself from the endless worrying that was haunting me. I spent hours distracting myself on Facebook. An old friend of mine, Val, sent me a posting on Facebook of a list of "25 things." It could be any twenty-five things you wanted. Twenty-five things you hated, you loved . . . anything.

I met Val in grade school and we remained friends throughout high school and college. She was one of my college roommates and my wonder twin. During high school we were a couple of lost souls, sulking around in black searching for our identity. Fearful that strangers would call us out on our dorkiness, ugliness, or strangeness, we stuck together - safety in numbers. We couldn't even walk into Circle K to buy our clove cigarettes without each other. All of our friends at the time had boyfriends. Val and I would sit in the park, smoking cigarettes and endlessly whine to each other, "Why don't WE have a boyfriend?"

Looking back I have to laugh thinking, "You were a big fat loser sitting in the park smoking, that is why you didn't have a boyfriend."

Later in college, Val found the boyfriend and I found boys. I dated, but kept far away from love. I was fearful of relationships. Fearful that if I fell in love they wouldn't love me back. Fearful of being hurt and rejected. I never let my wall down to reveal the real me. Although, I'm not sure I even knew who the real me was at that point. If I came too close to feeling strong emotions, or if they told me they loved me, my foot was out the door. Besides, who were they in love with? I never revealed the true me to any of them (any of them, except John.) I was well aware of what I was doing each time, but I couldn't help myself. No one cradled my fears or soothed my insecurities and my only defense mechanism was avoidance.

Val and I had kind of lost touch with each other until the dawning of Facebook. Now I always knew what she was up to and likewise. I loved reading Val's note. My initial thought was "No way am I doing that!" Val's writing was so stunning! Mine would sound so lame in comparison. Little by little, I started to think of my twenty-five things. I did indeed write my own note. I wonder had I done them a week earlier if they would have been the same.

Here is the note:

Holly's 25 things

Monday, January 26, 2009 at 3:09pm

Rules: Once you've been tagged, you are supposed to write a note with 25 random things, facts, habits, or goals about you. At the end, choose 25 people to be tagged. You have to tag the person who tagged you.

And, I won't be offended if you don't feel like doing this!

1. The best advice I've ever received was from my dear friend Julie. She told me, you need to find balance in your life. I did and it changed my world. Thank you!

2. I just realized last week I am a hopeless romantic. I love it all . . . the flowers, the notes, the sweet nothings, all the sap. True Love! It's what makes the world go around.

3. My favorite actors and actresses: Barbara Stanwyck - no one is gonna mess with her. Paul Newman - Hello!-- Hud should have been titled Stud. You can't

forget Betty, Joan and Bogart. I'm a sucker for the classics.

4. Favorite movies: Treasure of Sierra Madre - surprisingly not a Bogart romance. The Sound of Music - if only we could all sing our way through the day. Princess Bride - true love at its best. Mommy Dearest - the best movie quotes ever. Just to show that I do watch an occasional new movie - The Notebook - if John and I can go like this, we will be truly blessed.

5. Growing up I thought my Dad was strict. I now credit him with teaching me discipline, respect, honesty, loyalty, and integrity. If I can pass this on to our girls as well, I will be proud. I love you Dad.

6. My biggest regret was not asking my Grandmother her regrets before dying. I think she could have told me a secret or two about life.

7. I have a longing to give back. Laziness has held me back. I will be lazy no more.

8. I knew my calling in this life the day Hannah was born. I love being a mommy. I love you Hannah and Ivy!!!!

9. Julie also told me that you know you've found a good friend/mate when they can make you laugh like a thirteen-year-old schoolgirl. I have so many great friends. You know who you are. (Katie, I can't believe you didn't realize you were at the

top of this list.)

10. My favorite noise: Hannah and Ivy laughing uncontrollably. In fact I'm going to tape it.

11. My favorite food. Cheese!! Any kind, hot, cold, shredded, melted . . . Anything tastes better with cheese.

12. I have a strange fear of mustard and pickles. I'm sure a psychiatrist would have a heyday with this one. I believe it's actually attributed to my older sisters and their torture treatment.

14. No I didn't skip a number. I am extremely superstitious.

15. Like Val, I also worked at Phoenix Trap and Skeet pushing the button when the men with their rifles yelled "Pull." Even worse, was my job at Baskin Robbins. I ate ice cream everyday and got fat. I can't forget my most prestigious job as a cigarette girl in Las Vegas. I walked around with a tray of cigarettes, covered in tacky jewelry, working my light up yoyo, chanting "Cigars, Cigarettes, Yoyo's." What was I thinking!

16. I once broke up with a guy because he wanted to take me to the lake for the weekend. I just didn't want him to see me in a bikini. The fat feeling never left me even after the Baskin Robbins pounds did. I weighed 114 pounds at this time. If I weighed 114 now I'd be wearing my

bikini everyday . . . at the lake, the pool, the grocery store, school, any and everywhere. Sorry Eddie, I really did like you.

17. I'm amazed that I don't mind getting old. I don't mind the wrinkles, the grey, the few extra pounds . . . I've miraculously gained confidence with age.

18. There are a couple people I always hoped I'd run into again to say I'm sorry. I never thought I really would be able to until Facebook. Eddie, where are you? See 16.

19. My list wouldn't be complete with out mentioning John. I met him 17 years ago on the beach in Rocky Point. I think I fell in love with him that day and have been madly in love with him ever since.

20. I have many faults. I just don't like admitting them, not to you or anyone else. It's part of my OCD need for perfection. Damn, I just admitted one.

21. I tremble at the thought of having to speak in front of more than 5 people.

22. My favorite flowers are white spider mums. They always look like they're dancing.

23. I love to dance. I think I was reincarnated from the 50's/60's. I love to twist the night away.

24. Favorite Music: Wanda Jackson or any other good Rockabilly for that matter, Annette Funicello - That's right I said Annette. It doesn't get any happier than Annette. X/Knitters - John Doe's voice is almost as sweet as my hubby's, Johnny Cash - my Arkansas roots showing, and there has always been a little bit of a rocker girl in me. Rock on!

25. Cliché' it may be but I LOVE LIFE. I love the people, the smiles, the frowns, the moments, the sunshine, the sunsets, the sadness that only makes you appreciate the happiness, red toes, rainy days, giggles, purple, pop art, purple pop art, Hannah's new shoes, Ivy's stink eye, John's laughter, John's laughter with his brothers, John telling me I'm lovely, warm fuzzies, cuddles, family, and friends. I love it all.

26. I so enjoyed writing my 25 things.

Again, I can't help but wonder what my 25 things would have been just a few days earlier.

I received some of the most thoughtful responses to my 25 things. This note may have been what sparked me to write more in the weeks to follow. Some of the responses:

Valerie   That's beautiful, Holly! I remember in high school and college, threatening you with mustard and you would threaten me with worms!! I also remember very clearly, your comment when Hannah was born, that you were "made to be a mom" - it's great to see how much you love it and how good you are at it! And by the way - you have gotten more radiant with age!

<u>Nicole</u> Holly, You are the cutest person alive! I just read your list of 25 – I laughed and I cried. Gretch always says how darling you are. I couldn't agree more!!

<u>Vicki</u> You didn't need to include #25, because it's very evident you love life. More power to ya -- if only everyone loved life, we'd have world peace!!! You have a fantastic attitude and I'm glad we've reconnected!

<u>Holly Toner-Rose</u> Thanks Gals, You are both too kind. Val, I do remember Shelley and I threatening you on rainy days in your high heels with worms in 8th grade. Shelley was the troublemaker there.

<u>Shelley</u> Holly, I cracked up at the pickles and mustard. We always had to wait at McDonalds for them to make you a fresh "plain" burger. I also worked at Phx. Trap and Skeet. AND. . . I remember chasing Val with worms. What a brat...me, not you. You have always been sweet. These 26 things made me smile and laugh out loud.

<u>Jeanne</u> Holy Cow Holly! I loved reading your list. It has been the best part of my day! I guess I better start on mine. I could be up all night. Thank you for sharing.

<u>Leslie</u> You're such a fun and positive person!! So glad you're my friend and neighbor. Loved reading your 25 things!!

<u>Janice</u>   Reading your 25 things made my night. You are the best. We miss you.

<u>Gretchen</u>   You are so darned cute!! I got teary when I read about being a mama. You are such a good mam! Look at all the happiness shining through on your profile-pic!!! That's the best gift you can give those sassy sweet girls!!! Thank you for being you! Love, G.

<u>Holly Toner-Rose</u>   Gosh, I may have to write another 25 things just to hear some more of these wonderful compliments. Thanks gals.

Advice #5: Write your 25 things.

My worries kept coming, five days with my mind pounding in thoughts of doom, wave upon wave. Throughout this time, my first instinct was that I should go to church. Sitting in a church, with the stained glass windows, may make me feel safe and secure. I also saw one of John's scribbles that read, "Earn priesthood status". He must have thought the same thing. I'm not sure. I didn't ask. There is a little bit of background to this. Religion had been a source of strife in our relationship for years. John was raised Mormon and I was raised Catholic. Mind you, I have nothing against the Mormon religion and I don't believe John has anything against the Catholic religion. I was just raised Catholic and he was raised Mormon. Apples and Oranges, or my version is West coast/East coast - Both wonderful, just different. This was not a problem for us until we had children. Once we had children, like everything else, things changed. Now we had the issue of which religion to raise our children. I, of course, wanted to raise them Catholic and John wanted them to be raised

Mormon. So the arguments began. Catholic-Mormon-Catholic-Mormon. Neither one of us was willing to budge. We then came up with the idea to compromise and find an entirely new religion, so we went from church to church each week, shopping around if you will. Finally, we found one that we seemed to agree on, but after a while, I found that I was taking the kids to church by myself. If I was going by myself then couldn't I just go to MY church? And we were right back to Catholic-Mormon-Catholic-Mormon. John, at one point, insisted that the girls were going to be raised Mormon and I protested. Ensuing was the worst fight in our relationship. He threatened to leave me. Obviously he didn't, but what lingered was now a fear of speaking about religion. (This still makes me sad and I'm sure he feels the same way. But, what do we do?) We usually didn't discuss religion now, knowing what a touchy subject this could be.

So, with that in mind, my next thought immediately after "I should go to church" was, "No. That causes problems with John and me and we need each other more than ever right now. We need to be a unit. I don't think God wanted us to fight about which church to go to. I'm assuming that is not what He has ever intended. He put us together for a reason. We just need to pray. You don't need the stained glass windows or the priesthood status in order for God to listen to you." John and I have found a way to have God and spirituality in our home without having to go to a church. I think we would both like to go to church, and we would both love to make our parents happy by doing just that, but sometimes it just doesn't work that way. I do believe that Jesus has guided me through this, in fact carried me on a couple occasions.

I contemplated my death, more than several times, during those days of waiting. First I thought, "Ok, if this is the time for me to go, I can't complain. I have had a really great life. For seventeen years I have had true love in my life. I have two beautiful children whom I adore. I have no regrets. What more could I have wanted? If it's my time, I've lived a wonderful life. Truly wonderful! I'm okay with that.

WAIT!!!!! MY KIDS!!!!! They need me! Who is going to be there for them every moment? Who is going to teach them all the lessons they need to get through this crazy life? Who is going to be there? It needs to be Mommy. I can't leave them. God can't take me away from them. He just can't! I don't care about me, or my life, but this is their life! They need me! Who will be there to make it all better? Who will know how Hannah likes her food, how her idiosyncrasies are really gifts, know when she needs attention and when to pull back, know that when she pulls away she is really just hurt and scared - Who? Who will be able to read Ivy like a book and know when she is craving attention, but will never ask for it? Who will praise her as she dutifully marches on through her chores, homework, and more? Who will encourage all of Ivy's blossoming talents? Who will cheer them both on and teach them everything? I don't have enough time to do all this. God please don't take me! God please don't take me!!!!! And what about John? I need to be there for him. No one understands him like I do. He needs me. No one would treat him like I do, or love him like I do. He can't be alone in this life. God let me stay here with John. Don't take me away from him. I want to be there for him. I love him. He needs me. (I need him!!!!!!). He'll need a new wife. Oh God, he can't love her more than he ever loved me. I don't want him to have to be alone though. I don't want the girls to be without a mother figure. Oh God, what if his new wife just loves him for his money and doesn't love our girls? No, that wouldn't happen. John is very loveable. But she could love John and not love our girls. What if he marries some young bimbo and the girls think they need to be a bimbo too in order to get a man? Oh gosh! Don't take me God. They need me! What if his new wife wants to take my picture off of my huge picture wall? She just can't. I need to tell John that. The girls need to be able to remember me. Oh no, will they remember me?" (sobbing). "Okay, so his new wife can't take my picture down. She will just have to deal with my memory, but she can put new ones up of her. Ok, so John can marry one of my friends. They will keep my memory alive, love the girls, and love John as well. NNNNOOOOOO!!!!!!!! I want to be here to love John and love our girls (more sobbing). Please God! Don't take me from them, at least until the girls are eighteen. They will be okay after that. Wait, they will still need me through college and I want to be there to help guide them in relationships 'til they find the right man like I did. I want to send them little care packages and give them advice and be there when they need to cry. Okay God, please give me until the girls get married. They will be okay then. Wait! Having babies is so hard and changes your life so drastically. I want to be there to help them through that. There's so much I want to do for them. Please, please, please God don't take me 'til the girls get through the baby years with their children!! Oh God! I want to grow old with John. I don't want him to be alone. He would find someone who would love him quickly, but not like I would. I want to be by his side forever. I always dreamed that we would go together. God, I know you had guardian angels bring John and me together seventeen years ago, why would you take me away now? WHY? You can't do that. Please let me live. Please let me live!!!! (sobbing, sobbing, sobbing). You can't put us together and then take me away. Why would you do that??? Why me? Why me?" These are the horrifying thoughts that rushed through my brain minute by minute by minute.

I also spent a lot of time contemplating, "Why me? What did I do to deserve this? Was God punishing me for all of my sins? Did I not appreciate life that first week I found a lump? Why didn't I make a change then? Was God punishing me for that?" It just didn't seem fair. I have always been the kind of person who has stopped to notice the purple flowers. I had found the good in life, even when it was really bad. I noticed the rainbows, the smiles … I've said it all before. I appreciated life and mentioned it often. Maybe that was my problem; I was too vocal that I was happy in life and making others feel bad. Why? Why me? Was it that I was getting too confident? Damn that just wasn't fair! It took me thirty-nine years to find confidence. I'm confident I'm a good mom, wife and friend. It took a decade or two to overcome all of my insecure issues, and I had many of them. I'm even comfortable with my weight! I'm no longer 114 pounds, but I don't care. I'm in good shape, healthy - I feel good. Damn, that took some work to get there! Why are you going to take that away from me? All of it - Why????"

"Am I supposed to realize some calling from God that I haven't ever contemplated? Was this going to change my world? Was this supposed to change my world? What was my purpose here in this life? What?" I thought and thought and thought about this. In my mind I kept coming back to "MY PURPOSE IS TO BE A GOOD MOMMY TO HANNAH AND IVY AND A GOOD WIFE TO JOHN. Why then would God want to take me away?" I did have a nagging thought that I needed to give back more. That thought had been haunting me for a while. Every time I would comment on how happy I was, how lucky John and I were to have each other, how lucky we were to have Hannah and Ivy, how much we loved our neighborhood, our house, our backyard, our neighbors, our family, our friends, our girls having cousins . . . Every time I said something, I knew I should be giving back more to those not so fortunate.

Knowing a bit of our history will help you to understand our immense appreciation. John and I emotionally, had a storybook life for years. We traveled around experiencing adventure after adventure. On our first summer together, we drove to Alaska and worked in the fishing canneries for three months. We lived in a tent the first month on the banks of the Kenai Peninsula. We worked twenty hours a day, lived off of peanut butter sandwiches and smelled like fish, but life could not have been better. Later a fishing cannery hired us. It had dorm rooms with beds, hot showers and a cafeteria. These were all things we hadn't seen in a month, which made us feel like we were living in a palace. Every moment was a new adventure.

Our next stop was Las Vegas, Nevada. We both felt that Phoenix, Arizona was going to swallow us up. We were getting nothing accomplished there, and the city, the people, and our past were dragging us down. Wanting a fresh start and a new adventure, we packed up and moved to Las Vegas. While in Vegas, I chipped away at my college degree, and earned my money as a cigarette girl in the Casino. John was unsatisfied with the daily grind of 9 to 5 work. He realized he could make just as much money, if not more, buying records, antiques and vintage clothing from yard sales and thrift stores and reselling them to stores in Vegas. His business grew as we drove to California and Arizona to resell his goods there as well.

We lived very modestly during that time period and didn't want for much. Our house was the house, behind the house, behind the freeway, in the bad neighborhood kind of simple living. We recently drove past the "house" on a trip to Vegas with our girls (I'm surprised it has not been condemned or torn down). I told our girls, "This is where you will live if you don't go to college." The girls gasped at the sight. Funny thing is, never did John and I feel like we were suffering. We had each other, which equaled happiness in our eyes.

We figured if he could make money buying and selling across the states, why not take it, and us, across the whole United States. And so we did. The next summer we hopped in my car and drove back East. Our goal was New York City. We left Las Vegas with one hundred and fifty dollars. We financed our trip by stopping in little towns and purchasing "cool" clothes in thrift stores then heading to large towns and reselling them to vintage clothing stores. We made it all the way to Kentucky and ran out of time and money. I had to be back for fall semester. It didn't matter that we didn't get to New York. New York or New Mexico we were together.

On our long drive back home to Las Vegas we realized that we didn't fit into the typical mold of society. We never had. An inner voice screamed inside of us for independence. It may have stemmed from our strict upbringing as children and our rebellious nature or just our creative minds feeding off of each other - I don't know, but we had a dream to fulfill. We started to formulate our new plan. With a business proposal in hand we went to John's dad, Marv, to ask him for a business loan for our start up costs. He was very generous loaning us six thousand dollars to get us up and running. Within months of returning, we opened our first vintage clothing store together in Las Vegas, that we named "Recycled Rags".

We stepped it up a bit in the housing department, moving into the small apartment behind the store. We each worked four hours a day, if that. We didn't have a boss to answer to, no constraints on our time or material expectations beyond a car, food, and shelter. We truly had freedom.

Spontaneously, we would often pack a bag and a pile of cassette tapes and hop into our truck heading towards Cali. Endless weekends were spent in California accumulating goods for our store. We frequented unknown thrift stores in bad parts of town, yard sales in Hollywood with treasures from the past and huge warehouses with pile after pile of vintage clothing that we scavenged through. This was our enjoyment - our passion. We were like little kids searching for the golden treasure that only we knew about.

In one thrift store we frequented just beyond Barstow, Ca. we discovered a bag of key chains that read, "My job is great. People are good. Life is wonderful". We laughed so hard I just about peed my pants upon reading this because that was how we felt. For some unknown reason, we were given this key to happiness that no one else had. All of the people around us in life had a grimace on their face. Most of the people we knew in Vegas and back home complained about their spouse, their job . . . their life. We were lucky and we knew it and we laughed at how incredibly fortunate we were.

Every time we traveled to California, we felt like we had traveled home. We belonged there, so that is where we went. We sold our store and moved to San Diego where we opened another vintage clothing store "The Garage," right by the beach. We had the beach, our beach cruisers, and a little coffee shop next door. Who needed anything else? This time around we lived in the back of the store. It was very spacious (Not!) with a hundred square foot living room and a makeshift bathroom and shower. Our deluxe pad even included an upstairs loft - our bedroom. No matter that, in our bedroom we had to hunch over to avoid hitting our heads when standing up straight. It was our two-story beach paradise, and with all that, who needed a real kitchen? A hot plate propped up on bricks and a plank of wood worked just fine. I'm sure my parents must have been mortified at the places we lived. Looking back I am grateful for our adventurous, yet simple, life together. I would wish this upon our girls as well. We have the fondest memories of those years.

Everything changed when we had kids. Our girls were Irish twins, being born back to back. Hannah was just twelve months old when Ivy came along. We had two little babies to care for. When it was just us, we didn't care about the big house, the fancy car, fancy clothes, or anything else. Once we had kids, we wanted all of that for them. We wanted the house, the yard, the toys . . . Doesn't every parent? We at least wanted what our parents had offered us. To say John and I struggled once we had kids was the understatement of the year. While in California we worked night and day and then some to survive. We worked so much we didn't have time to enjoy our kids, or each other, much less the beach that we were paying ridiculous prices to be near. Our ideals of freedom and independence were suffocating us. The stress of it all had also been strangling our relationship. Engulfed in this intense stress, John resorted to drinking and I resorted to working. I worked harder and harder and John drank harder and harder. Not to say that one was better than the other, both were escape mechanisms. Resentment grew between us, and our relationship weakened day by day. We were penniless, loveless and just plain tired. To save our relationship and our family we threw in the towel and moved back to Phoenix. The move saved our marriage. I quit working 'til 2:00 a.m. and John quit drinking 'til 2:00 a.m. and our love rekindled.

We still had a few rough years after that assimilating to

the real world. We were still grasping onto our tired fantasy of freedom. Having been spoiled for years, working at our own business with no boss to answer to, it was difficult to think of joining the common workplace. The thought of having to report to someone else was horrific, for both of us, so we continued our business on the Internet. Our website was still doing well enough to survive and the emergence of Ebay brought about a whole new business for us. Financially, we still struggled. And we struggled. And we struggled some more. I remember having fifty-six cents in the bank and no food in the fridge. My sister, Sheree, showed up with a box of food from Costco and I cried. I cried in shame and in joy. Never had I pictured myself there. My husband decided to join the family business soon after that. I was very proud of him that day. I don't know if he realizes it, but he became a man in my eyes that day. He had always been my love, now he was MY MAN. He decided to give up his dream and provide for his family. I know this was hard for him and I'm still thankful for his sacrifice. Looking back now, I don't mind our struggling years one bit. I'm actually grateful that we went through them. I feel that is what has made me appreciate everything so much each day. For that I am thankful.

Long point made, I feel the need to give back to those that are still struggling financially. It gnaws at me. For years we couldn't afford to help anyone. We were the ones people were helping. Now we could afford to help out others less fortunate than us. "Why haven't we been doing anything?"

My husband would always tell me, "You help out so much at the school, that is your contribution."

I could never buy that. I knew that helping out at the girl's school was purely selfish. It benefited our girls and that was why I was there. I wasn't there out of charity. It was for our girls and our girls alone. "Granted, I'm sure it helps other kids and the school. But, come on, it's not charity. At least not to me."

Advice #6: Don't let anything hold you back from doing what is in your heart.

Chapter Four

Every day following my dreadful doctor visit seemed like an eternity. I don't know how many times I fell into John's arms, into his lap, or rolled over onto his chest. While sobbing I would tell him, "I'm scared! I'm scared John! I don't want to die. Don't let me die, honey!" I can't begin to describe how wonderful my hubby was through everything. I am truly blessed to have met him. Every time I had even winced a little, and more and more times sobbed, he stayed strong and positive.

He always told me, "You will be okay. You're NOT going to die, Holly. You are going to be fine." Each time he told me, I believed him. Every time he held me, I felt like he was holding me up. I can't imagine someone having to go through this without a wonderful supportive person. Thank you, John, for being my pillar and loving me so dearly.

I can only imagine what thoughts and emotions had been rolling through his head. There had only been a few times that I stepped aside to think about it. My newfound self-indulgence was difficult for me to accept. This was going to be a time in my life that I had to be selfish. I couldn't think about everyone else's feelings - not even John's. Worrying about me was all I could do. Not to say that I started walking around like a narcissistic maniac, I just had to focus on me to get myself through each day. I was not used to this, as my nature, I think, is to help other people and focus on others, or at least my family. I was having a hard time grasping this new characteristic. For the time being though, I was going to have to accept it. I had to put all attention on me.

Nights were the hardest for me. I couldn't keep my mind from racing to the "What ifs?" "What if I died? What would happen? What about the girls? What about John? What do I want at my funeral? Who will be at my funeral? What about my family? Crap, I still haven't told my family." The dark thoughts found me every night. They poked at me if I dared to fall asleep a bit. They are still the hardest.

We tried not to worry. We tried to keep things normal. To help us forget about cancer we surrounded ourselves with positive people. Laughter was our cure for the moment. John called his brother Danny, to see if he and his girlfriend wanted to go out to dinner. He is one of John's best friends. Danny is not only my brother-in-law, I consider him my friend as well. We met them for dinner and forgot all about lumps and doctors and the long hard road ahead of us . . . everything was normal for a couple of hours.

A few days later we were still trying to stay busy, busy, busy. John had told me how his mother sent around an email asking for everyone to fast on Sunday for me, and his sister Brenda, who was also having surgery that week. I was overwhelmed with emotions over this. It really was a blessed feeling to have all of these people praying for me and fasting for me. Every day I was crying thinking about the possibilities. Thinking about anything else was impossible. I had started to get a little testy with the girls. My patience was wearing thin. John was still strong. I tried to be strong.

> Holly Toner-Rose is thankful for her family! (and hungry)

Trying our best to stay distracted that morning, John read from the kiddie Bible, our newest attempt at having religion in our home, then we went for a Sunday drive, and next we went to the museum and then out to dinner with John's dad. By dinnertime we were starved, since we were fasting as well. We told our girls that we were all fasting for Brenda. Ivy's comment late in the day was "Why do they call it fasting? It's not even fast."

At one point during one of my hunger pangs my hubby said "Do you realize how many people are starving for you right now?" It was quite a few. John being Mormon had a large family. I cried thinking about how wonderful people were and how lucky I was. I then cried because I was scared.

Monday morning I received an early call from my sister-in-law Carol. Carol and I had spent a lot of time together over the past years and lived close in proximity. She is my sister-in-law and friend. We laugh, we cry, we complain . . . we do it all together. She asked me to come down to her tennis club, and do spa day since I had missed spa day with the girls. I was more than happy to accept. She was playing tennis 'til 12:00 but I was going to go there early and do my workout, sit in the jacuzzi and the wet spa (my favorite) until she was done.

On the elliptical, I ran like there was no tomorrow. I kept telling myself while running, "I will be okay. John's uncle said eighty percent are benign. I'm not going to die. I'm going to be okay." Faster and faster I ran. "Just one! Just one! I'm going to be okay. Just one!" Not being able to run my fears out of me, I decided to move on to something else. I lounged in the wet spa with the eucalyptus spray for an eternity. I stayed in until I thought I would pass out. I showered and then found Carol.

Advice #7: Spa Day!

Carol treated me to lunch and we sat in loungers soaking up the sun for what seemed like hours. I tried to figure out "the why?" with her. There seems to be a reason we go through some things in life. I think some events are God's way of teaching us lessons. Whether or not we gained from those experiences was up to us. "What was my lesson here?" I thought about what had changed. Fear, but that wasn't it. God didn't want me to live in fear forever. And I didn't think God had wanted me to die. I can't explain it but I just didn't feel he was going to take me, at least that day I didn't. John and I had changed. He instantly became the one I leaned on, the one I depended on. A few years back, it was the other way around in our relationship. I didn't care about the past, but John still did.

Maybe us having this experience would change things. He was taking care of me in every way. He became my solid rock. He was my handsome pillar. I admired him so for it. Maybe he could now let go of any anger or resentment he harbored towards himself for the past. Perhaps God was actually helping us.

I was able to share all of these thoughts with Carol. After the serious thoughts, we looked for the humor in it as well. Carol had always been the one to find comedy in any situation. Throughout the day, she continually made me laugh. She began calling it "Tha Caansuh" in her Grandmother's southern accent. She laughed that I now had an excuse for everything. I could blame anything I did or didn't do on cancer. She said just blame it on "Tha Caansuh." It was funny the first couple of times, but then the sound of "Cancer" started to creep in. I felt that as I kept hearing the word cancer, I was letting cancer inside of me. I didn't want to hear the word. I didn't want to have cancer. We laughed more about life, our kids, ourselves, . . . Everything. I hadn't been that relaxed in days. I was so appreciative.

Tuesday came and I still felt terrified. My tears had to be overwhelming for John by this time. I exercised that morning, hoping that would dissolve my tears and spark me on - it didn't. I went home and imprisoned myself to my house. The closet had been calling my name for a glorious self-pity session. I think every woman knows this feeling. Life's trials seem so much worse if you are crying in the closet, instead of crying in your room, or on the couch or anywhere else. It is the last resort. The worst of the worst, the "crying in the closet!" Being in the closet while crying, somehow validated just how dreadful it was. After my exhausting cry I grasped for a healthier option. I needed to escape my house, and my closet, so I made a small attempt to flee. My plan was to call my girlfriend Gretchen to see if she wanted to go have lunch. She never failed to make me laugh and I was confident I could open up to her.

Gretchen is another great friend. I became friends with her through my husband. He met her in Kindergarten and has stayed friends with her ever since. I'm so glad he did. Gretchen is an inspiration to me. She is a wonderful friend, mother, and wife. I remember the first time I spoke to her. She called John when we were living in Las Vegas, but he wasn't home. We got to talking, and an hour later, still on the phone with her, I felt like she was MY old friend calling to catch up with ME.

I called Gretchen and asked if she would like to go to for a late lunch. She nicely declined and then started to tell me what her crazy schedule was that day. She was in Target at the moment with her pseudo-adopted sons helping them get set up with all the necessities. It was just like her to be helping someone out. I wanted to jump in and say, "Gretchen, I may have cancer. I'm scared!" but I held back. I was on the verge of tears while talking. She must have somehow sensed this, because at the very end of the conversation she asked me how my doctor's appointment had gone last week. Being extremely emotional from the closet a few minutes earlier I couldn't keep the gates closed. I cried and told her it didn't go very well. I'm so blessed to have such good friends. She said "Oh my gosh! Oh my gosh! We do need to have a late lunch." Frantically she told the sons she needed to go. She said, "I'll be there in ten minutes. Go to my house and I'll be there." I don't think I argued one bit with her and I said I would be there. She dropped everything and came to my rescue that day.

For ten minutes or so I paced around the house and then drove over to Gretchen's. She lives in our Moon Valley neighborhood, just down the road. I walked up her walkway and before I reached the door she opened it and said "Oh you!" in her caring Gretchen way. She is like my hubby, in that, she has so many isms to her that are absolutely loveable. She opened her arms and just hugged me. I, of course, cried and she cried too. Sometimes a girlfriend's shoulder is all you need.

I cried and cried, recounting the story of the horrible doctor, who didn't show me one ounce of empathy. I told her how all I could think about was the girls. It all came down to them. As a mother, you didn't care about yourself. It was about your babies. John was on my mind as well, but the emphasis was on my girls. We talked about how 80% are benign and how I couldn't have cancer. It was just impossible. She told me John wouldn't let anything happen to me. And I was too happy of a person to get cancer. She asked me how I had been feeling physically. "Never better." I replied. I had increased my workouts in January and I had added hiking the mountain twice a week. Physically, I felt strong. She told me that she was so happy to hear that. Every person she knew that had cancer had said I just wasn't feeling very good. "That had to mean something! I was feeling physically strong. In fact the flu went around our house and I was the only one not to throw up. That had to mean something! Didn't it?" Her husband is a doctor and she told me she would ask her hubby to give me a call later to see if he could answer any questions. I just have to say "Thank goodness for girlfriends. They were all so wonderful to listen to me cry every week. Someday, I hope I can do something in return for them."

I left still thinking about my babies. I loved them so much. They were my life. I thought back to when my girls were teeny tiny babies and further back to being pregnant with them. A year after John and I were married we decided it was time to have kids. One week after we made that decision I found out that I was pregnant. We couldn't have been happier. I loved being pregnant and I loved my big huge belly. I didn't even care that I gained sixty pounds while being pregnant – well, maybe a little. I didn't care that I had to give myself shots everyday or I should say John gave me shots every day. My blood has a tendency to clot, since I have the minor blood disorder Leiden Factor V, and being pregnant increased this tendency. I had to give myself heparin shots while I was pregnant to ensure that my blood would not clot. Again, I didn't care. I was a proud mommy to be. We were still living in the back of the store with the hot plate, etc. We realized we needed more. We wanted a house, which we couldn't afford in

California, and we wanted our family near by, so we decided after Hannah was born we were going to move back to Phoenix and open another store there.

Hannah was born January 3rd, 1998. I had planned to have an epidural during her birth. I wasn't big on pain. The doctors gave me a big surprise when we arrived at the hospital. They informed me that there was too much heparin in my blood and I could not receive an epidural. Upon hearing this news I loudly pleaded, "TEST ME AGAIN!" I was in the most excruciating pain you can ever imagine. Every minute seemed like an eternity. The nurse came in two hours later and told me my blood was still too thin for the epidural. Again I cried, "TEST ME AGAIN!" Several hours later with no good news, a doctor offered me morphine to relieve the pain. Quickly, I accepted. I will never forget the nurse's words before she administered the drug.

"You will still feel the pain, but you won't care."

She was right. At some point later in the night I told the nurse, "I feel the pain and I care. Can I have some more?"

The doctors came in then, and told me "Good news. Your blood is okay for the epidural. Bad news is we've missed the window." Everything was somewhat cloudy after this since I was doped up on morphine. I didn't realize Hannah was too.

The doctor had me push and push and minutes later, out she came. All I saw was this huge grey cord twirled round and round - her umbilical cord. The doctor quickly snatched at something, fiddled with her mouth, and then threw the utensil back to the nurse. He screamed at the nurse for the next tool. I heard panic in his voice. "What was wrong with my baby? MY BABY!!"

Frustrated the doctor yelled out "THIS ISN'T WORKING! CODE 3!CODE 3!" All of a sudden a stampede of nurses and doctors ran into the room all hovering over my beautiful baby.

"What was happening?" Hysterical, I looked over at

John and he was as white as a ghost. A nurse told him he needed to sit down, that he was going to pass out. "MY BABY! OH GOD! MY BABY!" And then Hannah let out a cry. She had just decided to make a grand entrance.

For the next two weeks, I think we did nothing but stare at her with one of us on each side of her. We were part of God's creation with this magnificent little life in between us. She was our baby and a perfect little baby at that. We were a family. In the coming weeks I remember thinking, "I can do this. I'm good at being a mommy. This is my calling. Mommy!"

God had the perfect plan for us. Three months later, back in Phoenix, we found out I was pregnant with Ivy - Two little girls. We couldn't have been more blessed. I gave birth to Ivy on January 19th, 1999. With her birth, we planned things a little better, picking the date, so that I could have an epidural and skip drugging our baby and me on morphine. The doctor gave us four days to choose from. My sister Lorie and I looked at the astrological chart trying to figure out the best day. In the end John and I decided the 19th just felt right. So it was, January 19th, 1999.

We woke up early in the morning, kissed our baby Hannah goodbye, and told her we would be bringing back her baby sister with us and off we went. We arrived and they ushered us to a pretty blue room with butterflies painted on the walls. It was the perfect room for an innocent spirit to enter the world. The doctor came in and informed me that as soon as I felt pain to holler and they would give me the goods. Shortly after, I hollered and in they came. After the doctor administered the epidural I didn't feel an ounce of pain. John and I sat back hand in hand, watching Three's Company reruns on the TV. The doctor returned and told me that when I felt my next contraction to push. With a smile on my face I told him I didn't feel anything. The nurses had to watch my contractions on the monitor and tell me when to push. A few minutes later out popped my beautiful little Ivy. She screamed bloody murder the instant she came out. I heard her cries, "PUT ME BACK IN. IT'S COLD OUT HERE. I WANT MY MOMMY!" The moment they handed her to me she stopped crying. She was our brilliant little baby. She was perfect! Again, John and I stared in amazement at God's creation, of which we were so lucky to be a part. We returned home and this time we had Hannah staring over Ivy with us. Life was good. I loved being a wife, a mother and a family. I had found my place in this life.

Soon after Ivy was born John and I longed for California. We missed our life there and decided to try and make a go of it a second time around back in California. With Marv's help, once again we packed up our store, our house and our babies and went back to live the California dream. As I have mentioned already, this time around was no dream. It was more of a nightmare. For three long years we struggled. The dream died and our love was dying with it. We both agreed that to save our family we needed to get out of California. Life was too much of a struggle there. We couldn't handle the financial stress any longer. Back home we went to Phoenix. It was the best decision we ever made. There is not a day that I regret moving back to Phoenix. California would have swallowed us up had we stayed. No ocean breeze was worth our family.

Here I was, years later fighting for my family again, although this time around it wasn't financial stress I was battling, it was cancer. I didn't ever want to leave John and the girls. It was time for a little help from God. That night, before my appointment, my two brothers-in-laws were coming over to give me a blessing. This is a practice done in the Mormon Church. I must admit I have always felt at peace after I received a blessing. John's brother, Stephen, and Brenda's husband, Brandon, were there to give the blessing. I requested that Brandon give the blessing being that I was closer to him. John and I had lived with Brenda and Brandon in Las Vegas for six months or so on two different occasions. Let's just say they earned their place in heaven with that. Stephen started by anointing my head with oil. Brandon then spoke. When he first started speaking I couldn't keep the tears from slowly rolling out. I heard his voice waver a bit, which kept my tears flowing. Then midway through I felt a calmness come over me. I really did. My tears stopped. Brandon's didn't. I could hear the tears, the concern . . . the tender kindness eek out of him. I still felt calm.

I really do believe in the power of prayer. I don't care what religion you are: Mormon, Catholic, Baptist, Buddhist or simply a belief in God, God is listening to us all. I think it just requires a little faith and you can feel the Spirit. I sure did that day. I felt so calm.

Stephen and Brandon stuck around for a while and we visited. I didn't tell them at the time how I had felt the Spirit. I'm not sure if it was because I knew I would cry telling them, or if I just wanted to cling to the calmness for a moment longer. I did email thanking them a day or two later and described how I felt during the blessing and for a while after.

Advice #8: Pray.

Chapter Five

Wednesday, January 28th, 2009. John and I woke up super early to drive to Mesa, a neighboring city, for my biopsy appointment. We hadn't told the girls anything at that point. When leaving, we just said I had a doctor's appointment. Hannah had asked each time what it was for and each time I responded with, "I just have a regular checkup."

She inquired further with "ARE you SURE, Mommy?"

My mommy instinct kicked in and I reflexively replied, "Yes." She had always been a little too smart for her own good. She was piecing together our emotions, my doctor appointments . . . everything. I was happy that she bought my answer for the time being.

We drove to my appointment tense. Attempting to distract ourselves we listened to music. I was still trying to tell myself "Eighty percent are nothing." We nervously walked into the waiting area, signed in, and waited. We didn't have to wait too long.

They called my name, "Holly Rose." I asked if John could come in with me and the nurse said, "Not for this one. The rooms are just too small."

Forced to leave him behind, they escorted me to a little changing room. I was able to leave my belongings in the room and lock the door with a key. They ushered me to the next room. It was indeed small. It must have been approximately six feet by twelve feet. It contained a small patient bed with one twenty-inch monitor on a roll-a-bout with the attached machinery. As I lay on the bed, the nurse tilted me on my side with a small cushion beneath one side of my back. She proceeded to begin the ultrasound. She asked me where it was located on my breast, but before I could speak, she said, "Oh, there it is. I can see it."

I was thinking, "Crap! Is it THAT big? You can see it without even feeling for it. This can't be good."

Quickly, she did a brief ultrasound, identifying the area in my breast and then called for the doctor. The doctor entered with a smile. She was very nice and much more compassionate than the doctor at the first clinic, who told me I had a long hard road ahead of me. Before starting, she explained the whole biopsy procedure to me. While she performed her job she asked me about my life, my husband, and then about my kids. I was okay answering her questions 'til she asked about my kids. Tears started to roll out once more. "Just one! Just one! You can't ask me about my girls! It's all about them. I don't want to leave them. Just one!"

As she proceeded with the biopsy she explained each step to me. She showed me on the screen the needle being poked into my skin, then the miniature scissors inside of me on the screen cutting through my breast tissue, and then the minuscule vacuum sucking it out. It was really quite fascinating to watch. She said she would recommend to my ob/gyn that I have an MRI done. She added that sometimes she did that and sometimes she didn't. Before leaving she had me do one more mammogram. Afterwards, she informed me that the results would come back in twenty-four hours, so we would know if it was cancer or benign by tomorrow afternoon. The outcome could be life changing. The nurse ushered me back to the room. She said "Not to worry, you can just find a surgeon to schedule the removal . . ." I think she abruptly caught herself there and added, "If you need to get it removed at all."

John was the first person I noticed upon walking back into the waiting area. I was so happy to see him there. I had a sinking feeling in the pit of my stomach as we left the building. I squeezed his hand fearing the worst. As soon as we hit the parking lot I told him, "I don't feel good about this." I cried again. Poor John, he had to listen to my tears, yet again.

Once more, John consoled me, wrapping his loving arms around me. I cried. In the car, I held his hand tight and he held it back even tighter. I cried some more. Then I tried to be optimistic. "This is the best type of cancer to get, if you have to get it at all. You could just cut it right out. Odds are in my favor. Right?" I cried. John consoled. We went to lunch and sat on the patio. I recalled how the afternoon sun shining down on me at the spa with Carol had felt so good. I was hoping I could recapture the same feeling of relaxation. I didn't.

John made my next appointment for the MRI on Friday the 30th, two days later. I was hoping I didn't really need it, but my instinct at that point was telling me I had cancer.

Again, I thought about my girls. From day one they both brought me so much joy. Hannah was such a loving little girl and so bright. Her blonde hair and big blue eyes melted your heart. As a baby she wiggled across the floor full of giggles, bringing so much happiness into our lives. She reminded me so much of myself, but she was so much better. God took my practical brain and my compassion and added John's intelligence and wit resulting in a perfect combination - Hannah.

At age three she was problem solving for me. A chair would break and she would tell me "Mommy you can just fix that. If you take my sippy cup and push a straw into the hole and then attach three more straws, one by one, and glue Ivy's rattle onto the end it and put the rattle into the bracket it will be all better." Funny thing was, she was always right. Had straws been able to hold up the weight of the chair, it would have worked. Her mind was always going. She would also tell these fantastic detailed stories with such exclamation in her voice, animation in her face, and gesticulations that you wanted to hear more, "And THEN the EEEEEEVIL giant came around the corner ..." At age eleven her stories rivaled those on our book shelves. She was writing her name by the time she hit three and she was drawing me picture after picture of seahorses. She is extremely empathetic. She always notices if people are happy, sad or angry and wants to make them feel better if they are the latter. She was always giving me loving cards pouring out what a good mommy I was in crayon and still does. I'm so thankful she received John's witty gene. She always keeps us laughing. She can keep up with any adult conversation. In fact, if there's a playful banter, she will most likely top all responses. She is so smart. She can't talk fast enough to keep up with the thoughts that are churning in her brain. I've always explained things to her, as I would to an adult, not like a child, even as a baby. I sensed she understood somehow. I know that sounds odd, but I swear she understood. She would give me knowing glances and look at me differently acknowledging she comprehended. Maybe it is just that our minds are so similar. We are both always organizing, projecting what will happen next, thinking of a better way to do something, imagining, inventing . . . dreaming. Never do we do anything half way. If you are going to do something - you do it right. This was my dad's motto and also mine and now it was Hannah's. I anticipate that when we she grows up we will both appreciate our similar qualities in each other. We'll forever be friends. I love her so much.

And I thought about my Ivy. Ivy is so sweet and innocent. She reminds me so much of John as well. Not only does she look like John with her big green eyes with flower petals in them, she carries his charisma. You can't help but be taken in by her. Even watching her eat is somehow fascinating. When she was little she did everything with a whimsical attitude. She was the epitome of innocence.

A few years ago she came to me and said "Mom! Hannah told me Mickey and Minnie aren't real. They are just people dressed up in costume. I don't believe her!" She was nine at the time. She loved the fairytale idea of life. For two years she dressed up as a different princess everyday, actually make that five different princesses everyday. I think she may have even convinced herself she was a princess. One of Ivy's preschool keepsakes is a picture of herself with the caption she wrote, "I'm special because my hair is sparkly." It wasn't really sparkly. She just wanted it to be, so she made it true in her own eyes. That was my Ivy. Innocence and happiness. Her artwork captures her soul. Every picture she draws is filled with smiles. Her pictures never fail to brighten my day. She is also graced with her daddy's athletic gene, mastering every sport she tries with ease. She is so strong and courageous, just like her daddy. She marches on dutifully with her homework and chores. She is also fearless and never afraid to put herself out there, to try something new and different. She is not afraid to fail. She takes those moments as practice or as stepping-stones, to acquiring new skills. I'm so proud of her. She is always honest and open with her feelings. In fact, I often get her opinion if I was too hard in my discipline. She will quickly tell me, "Mom, I don't think Hannah deserved a time out." And she'll tell me why. She is usually right. We all laugh that she is the keeper of time. Every morning I hear, "Hannah, it's 7:32, we have to go. Hannah, it's 7:35, we're going to be late. Hannah, it 7:36, we need to leave now. HANNAH, it's 7:39. Hurry! HANNAH, IT'S 7:40! I'M LEAVING." It's really part of her integral compass. She does what is right. She is on time, follows the rules, sticks up for herself and others around and expects everyone else to do the same. She is a role model. She will forever be my baby. I love her so much.

When I returned home from my biopsy appointment I called a few close friends. My dear, friend Julie - I love her. She is my girlfriend from Las Vegas. She is my conscience. During our struggling years in San Diego after our children were born, she was my main emotional support. Her long talks helped to keep my and John's marriage afloat. She has always been there to listen and gave me uplifting advice. She is a special person who radiates a bright shining light. I believe God has a special calling for her.

I also called my girlfriend, Katie. She is considered family. My girls call her Aunt KK. I think she is one of the smartest people I know. She has achieved so much in her lifetime. I am proud of her as a person and as a friend. I love her.

Katie and I became close friends in the sixth grade. We

spent our grade school summers together having sleepover after sleepover. During those summer months we stayed up late watching Dawn of the Dead (that led to her adult preoccupation with Zombies) and Vacation endless times, we created magnificent water ballet acts in the pool, snuck out of the house to toilet paper the neighborhood boys' houses, learned Michael Jackson's dance moves by heart (I still know the dance and I bet Katie does too) and laughed our heads off at the silliest things. High school came and as the years ticked by we started to drift apart. We both found new friends. Even though we were all interconnected we were no longer best friends.

We went our separate ways going to different colleges, but kept in touch. Our friendship somehow grew stronger hundreds miles away from each other and we have maintained our bond ever since. Boys and college and trips and work and money (or no money) and babies, none of it ever severed our friendship, nor do I think anything ever will. Our friendship is something I treasure.

I can't recall whom else I called. I still hadn't called my family. I was telling myself at this point, "No need to worry them."

That night I got down on my knees and prayed to God. I had been praying all along, but I don't think I had made it down on my knees. I said the Lord's Prayer. "Our Father who art in heaven . . ." I don't know how many times. This prayer had always brought me comfort. Anytime I was scared, felt an evil spirit, felt temptations, mean spirited thoughts . . . you name it, "Our Father" took everything away and left me with a sense of peace. I said "Our Father" some more. Ending with "Please, Dear God don't take me away from them. Don't take me away from John and the girls! I really do want to live. I want to live! I love them! And love living! I'm begging you. Please!" I prayed for forgiveness of any sins I had done in the past. I prayed for survival. I prayed.

Thursday, January 29th, 2009. This was the longest day

of my life. The results of my biopsy were coming in that day. That day I would find out if I did have cancer. The girls went off to school as normal. I tried my best to keep busy. Every time the phone rang my heart stopped. "This is going to be the call. They are going to tell me I have cancer." Ring ring. "This is going to be the call." Clean, clean, Ring ring. Sob! Sob! Hour after hour dragged on. "This is going to be the call . . . I CAN'T TAKE THIS ANY MORE! Why don't they just call? WHY? WHY?" I fell into John's arms again and again in tears. My strength had disappeared. As the phone kept ringing, I told John I wasn't taking any calls that day. I couldn't speak to anyone but John. Shelley called, Lisa called, and Katie called. One by one friends called and John had to inform them what was going on. He also told them I wasn't talking to anyone.

I kept myself busy Facebooking half of the day. At one point, I posted on Facebook, what I thought was inconspicuous about my status.

> Holly Toner-Rose is waiting not so patiently.

I received a few responses with suggestions to keep myself occupied:

> Carol Holly, get soduko book and hang in there. Did they tell you how long you would have to wait????

> Carol P.S. I have no idea how to spell Soduko... or how to do those.

> Stacie What are you waiting for?

> Carol P.P.S. A really fun thing to do while waiting is to go to the Bad Plastic surgery website. I enjoy it, anyway. XXOO

> Alisha Holly, Watch episodes of 30 Rock or The Office.

Time stood still. Ring, ring. Heart stopping. John answered "Hey Katie". Sob, Sob.

That repeated itself through out the day. "WHY? WHY? WHY was this taking so long? They said twenty-four hours! Oh my Gosh! I HAVE CANCER! I CAN'T HAVE CANCER!!!! WHY DON'T THEY CALLLLLLLL!!!!!!!!"

The girls came home and still no news. Homework. Clean, clean. Sob, sob. The girls had tennis that afternoon and Hannah and Ivy were ready to go. I heard the phone ring again. Then I heard John close his office door. "Oh God! This is it. They are going to tell him I have cancer. I'm not ready. I'M NOT READY!"

"JOHN, I'm taking the girls to tennis!" I quickly grabbed the girls and ran out. I dropped them off at the club just down the street and drove back. Trying to gain my composure, I took in a deep breath, another deep breath, and then another.

"Oh God. John is going to have to tell me I have cancer. Why? Why? Oh God." Deep breath. "Okay. I can do this. I can do this. I'm ready."

I walked in the door, and slowly walked towards his office. "Oh God, the door is still closed. What if he is in there crying? Oh God! I have cancer!" I slowly opened the door and he was sitting at his desk, like usual. I'm sure I had a blank expectant stare. He didn't say anything. "Oh God! I have cancer!"

Trembling I asked him, "What did they say?"

John calmly replied, "He said the results won't come in until tomorrow." Like a little baby, I broke down sobbing once more. I think this was truly the weakest moment I had ever experienced in my lifetime. My body shaking, I sobbed more in his arms. He held me tight. He kissed me, and said, "Everything will be fine Holly." I felt strong again for a brief minute.

Shelley called back sometime after this. She demanded to John to have me pick up the phone. She wasn't going to accept no for an answer. I took her call. I was happy that I had so many people from my childhood still in my life. Shelley and I became friends in the sixth grade. Back then she was very outspoken and I was super shy. Shelley was loud enough for the both of us, which helped hide my awkward shyness. She was always super funny and I was always ready to laugh at her jokes. We were a mischievous pair. She was the mastermind and I was the eager helper ready to carry out the plan. We were a couple of pranksters that laughed and giggled our way through grade school. Thirty years later, Shelley and I both had our different circles and different lives yet we were still intertwined and I'm guessing, forever would be. She is a wonderful person and friend.

On the phone Shelley told me how, four of her friends she knew just found lumps and all came back benign. "Crap!" I thought, "One in four is cancer. That means my odds just went down." We talked for quite a while. It felt good talking to another woman and releasing some of my fears. Poor John had already gone through hell and back listening to me cry. Shelley asked at the end of our conversation to post something on Facebook, so she would know what the results were. That way, she wouldn't have to bother John or me by having to make a bunch of phone calls. I liked the idea.

I called Katie, Julie, and Gretchen and said, "No news, so not to worry. Have fun tonight and I'll call you tomorrow."

I hung up the phone and poured myself a glass of wine to try to calm my nerves. Then I searched for John. He was in our bedroom ironing his shirt. I plopped myself down on the bed. He told me he was going to get out of the house for a bit. I was happy for him. He needed a break from all of this chaos. And besides, we weren't going to find out until tomorrow.

As I sat watching John, I shared with him that it was the waiting that was the hardest part. I couldn't wait any longer. I told him "If they could just tell me, I can deal with it. I just

61

can't handle waiting any longer. It's killing me."

He looked at me so lovingly, with his shirt in his hand and calmly said "Holly, it is cancer." His voice was melodic. I'm not sure why I say that. I think that it was the love that poured out of him in those few words. He loves me so.

After he told me, I know I cried, but that time softly. I had cried too many tears that day. My fear had been exposed. I did sense some kind of peace just knowing. I was ready to battle this. I could do this. If any person could beat cancer, it was me. I could always find the positive. That was my forte. I could find the strength to fight. I could do this. I would be okay.

John went out for a couple of hours. He needed it. My dear, dear hubby, he never showed me one tear. I'm so thankful that he didn't because I would not have been able to handle it. Thank you John once more for your strength and love. I still can't believe you walked around our house for a half an hour or so keeping it inside of you. You are the strongest man I know. I admire you! I love you!

While John was gone, I made my post on Facebook, for Shelley and the few others waiting to hear, my results:

Holly Toner-Rose is ready to fight!!!!

I figured that was pretty indiscreet. That could have been applied to anything. I could have been fighting with a neighbor or fighting with John . . . Anything, or so I thought. I think Katie was the first to respond.

> Kate Holly - You're going to fight and you're going to beat it! You can be pretty darned determined when you put your mind to something!
> xoxo
> Kate

> Shelley Holly...you know you can do it! You're not alone...we're all here to help!

Janice Holly, We love you! Stay positive and strong and kick some a_ _. We are here for you.

Valerie Holly, who or what are you fighting??

Vicki You have such a great attitude. This is a fight I KNOW you will win.

I then decided to call Julie and Katie. Having just gone through the torture of waiting, I knew it was the hardest part, and I didn't want Katie or Julie to have to go through that either. I called Julie first. She is a great friend to me. I miss her. I miss her funny stories, her laugh, her bright light . . . I wish she were near so my daughters would be influenced by her as well. She is such a positive, honest person with a good soul. I called and told her the news. I have no idea what I said or what she said. I know she made me feel better. She always did.

Next was my call to Katie. I immediately got to the point and told her I have breast cancer. We cried together. She said I would be fine. I agreed. I'm confident she made me laugh somehow, like she always did. Not sure what else we said. I love her dearly. I'm so thankful that she had recently moved back to Phoenix, Arizona from Barbados. (She had been living/working in Barbados for the past two years.) She has been my strongest supporter through all of this, with the exception of John of course.

I hung up the phone and she immediately called me back crying and told me I had to promise her something. I asked her what? She said, "You have to promise me that you aren't going to die." I knew exactly how she was feeling. We had very similar personalities, both being Capricorns. I think we both always tried so hard to be strong, perfect and independent, but sometimes we just couldn't do that. At that moment I couldn't be strong for her. I told her I wasn't going to die, but that she couldn't do this to me. I asked her if she wanted Julie's number. She said, "Yes" and I gave it to her. They could cry together, but not to me, at least not just yet.

Again, I was learning I had to be selfish. That is something I wouldn't have done to Katie a week ago. I would have buried my feelings and tried my best to make her feel better, but right then, I just couldn't. It was all I had in me to get myself up, put on a smile and get myself through the day. I could do no more.

I still hadn't told my family yet. "Why worry them 'til we know more? I might as well wait until we see the surgeon. Right?? I'll wait a bit longer." But, I knew deep down why. They were going to be the hardest to tell.

John came home and we hung out with the girls the rest of the night. We did "lay time" in Hannah's room. "Lay time" consisted of about one hour most nights. We would lay together as a family and John would read to us, or we would play a game, or I would just watch John wrestle with Ivy, calling her Chavalita, and her jokingly come back with "Get your man boobs off of me you big gorilla," while Hannah told me stories, or we would all just talk about our day. I'm not sure when we started this. I think even when they were babies we did this. It was our evening tradition that just seemed to stick in our family. It was a tiny bit of time with no TV, no computer, no iPod, no phones, and no cell phones . . . Nothing. It was just us connecting as a family. We used to do this around five times a week and it seemed that lately it had dwindled down to tops, once or twice a week. I made a mental note that we needed to change that. I missed it. Our girls missed it. We only had a couple of years left with them 'til teenage years kicked in. After that we guessed they would be too cool to want to hang out with us. They just turned ten and eleven. (We're still crossing our fingers that won't be the case.)

I thought back to all of the wonderful times we had with our girls. It would be a sad day when they no longer wanted to hang out with us. When Ivy was a baby she only wanted Mommy. If anyone picked her up besides me she would scream and scream bloody murder. She was such a finicky baby that even if she was fast asleep and someone moved her thumb, she would wake up screaming, "WHO

MOVED MY THUMB? WHO TOUCHED ME? WHO?"
Then, if she saw that it was me, she would instantly calm
down. Anyone else, she kept screaming just to let you know,
"DON'T EVER TOUCH ME AGAIN! YOU ARE NOT MY
MOMMY!" We tell her that now and she laughs and laughs.
She was so content in my arms for years. She sucked away at
her thumb without a care in the world. She didn't want to grow
up. When I would ask her, when she was a few years older,
what she wanted to be when she grew up she would flat out tell
me, "I don't want to grow up. I want to be a kid forever." She
wasn't stupid. She knew what being grown up entailed and she
wanted to have fun.

Hannah was the opposite. She loved everyone as a
baby. She would let anyone hold her and everyone wanted to
hold her. She never cried, never screamed. She was as happy as
could be. She loved her baby sister Ivy. Hannah couldn't
pronounce her V's so she called her I.G. She was always super
protective of Ivy and constantly checking to make sure Ivy was
okay. She would hand her bottles, food, wrap her in blankets
even if it was 115 degrees out. At the park she would stop
every couple of minutes and look to make sure Ivy was safe. I
think she'll forever do that. I'm happy they have each other.
They will always have each other for comfort I thought – just-
in-case.

That night I had a dream. I had always been a big
believer in dreams. A few times I believe that God had given
me messages in dreams. Once about finding my faith again,
once about my grandfather, Philip, who passed away, once
when my sister Lorie was having problems, and again when
John and I were struggling in our marriage over religion.
Sometimes they were clear as day, and sometimes I had to try
to decipher them. It may sound like hogwash, but I believed.
Faith!

So here was my dream. Take it for what you want. I
was in the backseat of a car driving down the road at night.
John was next to me. I'm not sure who was driving. The

window was rolled down just slightly. I could see in the corner of my eye a black figure walking up. He was covered in menacing burglar gear: black pants, black long sleeve shirt, black ski mask, black gloves . . . the works. He reached his arm in the slit of the window grabbing around frantically for my purse. The car started to take off and I saw my little black, fringed bag go out the window with his arm. The car sped away and left the burglar behind. I looked down and saw my big purse there in the car. I was relieved that he didn't get my purse. Everything important I had with me was in my purse. My little pretty fringed bag just had some makeup inside. He didn't get anything that I couldn't replace.

The next morning John drove me back to Mesa for my MRI. I relayed my dream to him. Here was my interpretation. The burglar was cancer trying to rob me of my life. Cancer wasn't going to take my life though; it was just going to take a snippet of time from me. I was going to be okay. It wasn't going to take anything important from me, just a little vanity, maybe my breasts, maybe a few scars, maybe my hair . . . I didn't care. I was going to be alive with my girls and with John. That day I felt good. I was going to be okay. That was all that mattered.

On the way there, the doctor's office called and left a message on my phone and said the MRI machine was broken and I needed to reschedule. We were five minutes away when we received the call. In unison we cried out "Let's say we didn't get the message, let's throw a fit." We realized we weren't eighteen any longer. There was no need to lie, nor did we want to lie. Who needed bad Karma at this point?

We walked up to the counter and the woman said, "Oh, they fixed it. No need to worry, everything is on time." We were both very thankful.

They called my name again. I followed once more to the little room, changed into my gown, took my key and followed the nurse to a new room. This was a large room with the MRI machine. MRI stands for Magnetic Resonance

Imaging. The machine uses a powerful magnetic field, radio frequency and a computer to produce detailed pictures of the inside of the body. This allows physicians to better evaluate parts of the body. The MRI machine looked like an enormous futuristic white rocket lying on its side with a hollow center. In front of the machine stood a fancy looking patient bed, contoured to fit body parts.

The two women present were both very cheerful. Nicely, they explained what was going to happen. They told me that the bed I was going to lie on would move into the hollow tube. They would leave the room, but would have contact with me via headphones if there were a problem. An initial series of scans would be taken. One of the nurses would reenter and insert something into my IV that would produce a contrasting image for the second series of images that would be taken. I would have a pair of headphones to listen to music throughout the procedure.

The nurses assisted in positioning me correctly on the bed. I lay on the table face down with my head propped in between foam cushions, similar to those when you have a massage. My head was then strapped in to help prevent me from moving. They moved my breasts this way and that into cushions of their own. Satisfied with my placement, one nurse told me they were ready to roll.

She emphasized to me, "No matter what, DON'T move. We need every image to be exact to be accurate."

I said, "Okay." They asked if I was comfy and I said, "Yes."

The machine turned on and my bed inched its way into the space age mechanism. I could hear one of the two nurses on the headphones. She softly said "Okay. This one will be about 2 minutes." Then the music tapped in.

All of sudden I heard "Baaahhhh!, Baaaaahhhh!, Baaaaaahhhh!" I felt like I was in the middle of an air raid and the warning sirens just sounded. "Baaahhh!, Baaaaahhh!

Baaaahhhhh!"

"Holy crap! This is really happening to me!"

"Baaaaaahhhh! Baaaaaahhhh! Baaaaaaahhhhh!"

Then the soft tone came again. "This one will be about 4 minutes."

"Baaaaahhhhh! Baaaaahhhhhhh! Baaaaahhhhhh!"

"Oh no! Just one! Just one! Just one! This is too surreal for me! Just one! Just one! Just one!"

"Baaaaaahhhh! Baaaaaahhhh! Baaaaaaahhhhh!"

Gentle voice, "This one will be about 6 minutes."

"Baaaaaahhhh! Baaaaaahhhh! Baaaaaaahhhhh!"

"Holy Air raid coming! I can't do this! I'm not strong enough for this! Damn it!"

Baaaahhhh! Baaaahhhhh! Baaaahhhhh!

"My forehead hurts and I can't move."

"Baaaaaahhhh! Baaaaaahhhh! Baaaaaaahhhhh!"

"I need to move. My forehead is in pain."

"This one is about 4 minutes"

"Baaaaaaahhhhh! Baaaaahhhhhh! Baaaaahhhhh!"

"I DON'T WANT TO HAVE CANCER!!!!" And then it was over.

The women helped me out and I asked them if I should find a surgeon at this point. One of the nurses told me, "You don't even know that it is cancer yet. You go home and have a good weekend and wait for the results first."

I informed her that I had already found out that it was indeed cancerous. "Now should I find a surgeon?"

She chuckled. Her last words were, "If it were me, I would just have them both cut off and get new ones. They will be perky 'til you are 90." We both laughed. I went and changed back into my clothes and found my hubby once more.

We drove home and I think we both found positive things that time. "I could get new big boobies that would be perky 'til the day I died. If you had to get cancer I got the best kind to get, didn't I? You could just cut it right out. We found it early. Thank goodness for Shelley and her Facebook posting." I felt good. I could fight it. I wasn't going to sit back and do nothing now.

Returning home I remembered this story that came out during my college years. A young boy found out he had a brain tumor. He imagined all day that his brain tumor was an asteroid, like in the video game, and he kept mentally firing at it. He did this twenty-four/seven. Later, back at the doctor's office they said his tumor was gone. It was a miracle and unprecedented! It just plain disappeared. When I read this story in college, I told myself to remember this. I believed that there were untapped areas in the brain that had more power than what we actually used. So here I was, with breast cancer some twenty years later. I was going to do the same thing. Or at least I thought that for a brief second. I acknowledged very soon that to focus on one thing for that long is nearly impossible. I also realized that I was so busy trying to keep myself distracted from the thought of cancer, that I couldn't play asteroids on my cancer and not think of my cancer at the same time. At night when my thoughts flooded me about cancer, I was usually praying for God to keep me and why. A few times, I tried to focus and kill the cancer with my superior brain energy, but I couldn't do it for long. More power to that little kid. I thought to myself, "I think I may need the help of modern medicine."

That afternoon I logged onto Facebook. By then, I had many concerned messages about what was happening to me:

> Jeremy Holly, is everything okay?!?
> ~michelle

> Emily Hey sweetie! I'm thinking of you
> and saying some prayers . . .

Anna Holly, We are thinking of you!

Alissa Holly--I'm not sure what you're going through, but I'm sending you a super lot of warm thoughts and bright wishes to wrap around you...

John was getting postings on his Facebook as well, and phone calls started coming in all worried about me. I realized that people had figured out something bad was happening to me, some just not sure what. To cease everyone's anxiety I had to post something on Facebook. I must admit, it was pleasing to see the concerned postings to my wall coming in. Each and every posting picked me up, every time. I don't think I intentionally ever thought, "I will tell everyone and be upfront about this." I just did. Maybe it was my way of getting through it. Maybe I knew I needed the extra emotional support. I wouldn't have expected that of me. If someone asked me a year ago what I would do in my situation, I would have said I would only tell a few select people. Now, here I was telling people I hadn't really spoken to in twenty years. I'm so pleased that I did share my news with everyone.

Here is the note I posted: "I will win!!!"

I will win!!!!!

Friday, January 30, 2009 at 1:16pm |

So my encrypted message on Facebook to a few in the know was not so cryptic. As you have probably figured out by now, I just found out I have breast cancer. I have to say a big Thank you to Shelley for sending me the posting on Facebook reminding me to perform a self-check. It may have just saved my life. For all of you ladies on Facebook you will be receiving a reminder email from me every

70

month. As we all love to escape on Facebook for fun, I promise to keep my postings a little more on the bright side. We will post notes with details on progress on my page for those that are interested (Scroll down on the left side and click notes). At this point the biopsy taken tested positive for cancer. The doc said it is small (again thanks Shelley) and lucky me I have big boobies so they think they can save it and if they can't I get brand new and improved boobies. I just did a MRI this morning so the doctors will know exactly what they need to take out. As soon I we get the lumpectomy scheduled, we will post the date.

I have to say thank you to everyone for the wonderful notes of encouragement and prayers. It is very uplifting to me, and to John. I am so thankful for you all. You all made me cry with happiness. I have no problem saying keep them coming!!! And if you are friends with my wonderful hubby send them his way as well. He is my pillar, as you all know. I know they lift his spirits too.

I do want to say that I feel very good about everything. The hardest part, was not knowing. Now that I know, I know I'm going to be o.k. I just have a little fighting to do. If anyone can fight cancer it's me. I've got the fiery red headed spirit in me and they don't call me Hollyanna for nothing.

Thank you again for your love and

support. Love, Holly

Responses on Facebook poured in:

Alisha You are amazing Holly! We know you will beat this and encourage us all at the same time.

Vicki God bless you! I'm so happy that you seem to have found it early. You're so wonderful and I've really enjoyed getting to know you again. You're absolutely right -- you WILL win. I know it. I hope we can still get together for some hikes. Most importantly, though, take care of yourself. Love,
Vicki

Jeanne Your positive attitude is great! You will win! Remember that we are all here for you, John and the girls, so whenever and whatever you need, just say and we'll be willing to help! We will keep the prayers comin' and fight along with you! Love to you and the family!

Jeremy Holly, I am so sorry to hear about all of this!!! You are going to be fine, you are a very strong woman, you CAN beat this!!!!!!! If there is anything you need please do not hesitate to let me know. I am NEVER to far away to help a friend. Thanx for the post and I will be looking for all the updates on your progress. Much love being sent out to you and to yours. You are in my thoughts and in my prayers!!!!! Love you~M

Carol B. Holly, your letter was an inspiration. If anyone has the fighting spirit and optimism needed, YOU ARE

THE ONE!! Our family is stronger and better because of you! We love you. You are in our prayers all day!

Valerie Thank you Holly, for being an inspiration to us all. You are so loved by so many! We will all keep our support and love and prayers coming. And thank you Shelley, for sending that post around!

Kate If anyone can beat this, it's you! And, there's nothing wrong with being a "Hollyanna", especially when you have the strength (of body, mind and spirit) to turn the positive thoughts into positive results!
I think Carol said a mouthful when she said that her family is better for having you in it! I know my life is better for having you in it (and I have no intention of NOT having you in it for a very, very long time).
I love you!
Kate

Eric I hereby donate all the rest of my redheaded spirit to you as we reds need to stick together. Keep up the good fight. Let me know what we can do.

Emily Oh Holly! I know you will win! You and John are two of the strongest (not to mention funniest, warmest, silliest) people Stuart and I know. We are thinking of the two of you and the girls and sending lots of love your way..........

John You're damn right you will win! We won't let you lose.

H. Shelton We love you all & will

73

continue to keep you in our thoughts & prayers. Please do not hesitate to call if you all need anything at all. Friends are for leaning on in your time of need & it sounds like you have a lot to lean on if you need to.

John Rose Ever seen The Legend Of Billie Jean? At one point she cuts off her hair like Joan Of Arc. I'm half-expecting Holly to do the same (or at least tie a bandana around her wrist) as Pat Benatar plays in the background.

Jennifer Big Big Big hugs being sent your way from San Diego. My first thought is of your beautiful daughters. I can see that your strength and optimism is going to help them through this as well

Carol Never doubted it.

Kate Holly - you need a theme song!

Anita I am with you all the way for everything that you may need! I love you and I am thinking of you! I hope to see you soon, I still have your Birthday present in my closet!!!

Curt Damn right you will win -- no doubt in my mind. We'll send you good thoughts from over in Germany, so you know the whole globe is with you ;)

Monica Go get'em! Wolverine Pride! You are in my prayers-Monica

Ruth You'll be in my prayers.

Marina John and Holly, you two will be in our prayers! Hey, if you can live with

John in that cramped "house" in back of The Garage in P.B., you can get through anything! :)

John Rose Marina. I don't know why people always make jokes about our "house" in P.B. It had a working shower, a hot plate, and (sort of) a loft. So what if you couldn't stand up straight in the upstairs makeshift bedroom?

Gretchen Oh Holly Holy!!!! I so love you!!! I am here for you always!!!! The power of a positive mind is so fantastic! That is why you will WIN!!!!! Anything I can do for you, John or the girls you please let me know!!!
Love, Gretch

Nicole Thinking of you. You are a Strong, Bright light, w/ amazing strength! Sending you a big hug. Go, Holly, Go!!

Christopher Love you, I know that your spirit and drive will overcome this.

Jerry Holly...You'll be in my thoughts and prayers. I can't believe how brave you are. Truly an inspiration. I know you will beat this. All my best,
JR

I'm not sure I can even begin to describe how touched I was by each and every posting. I felt like I had the whole world behind me. How could I possibly lose with John, my friends and my now my entire Facebook network on my side? Lucky me. I was going win!!!!!

Advice #9: Share with your entire network that you have cancer. The support you receive from every last person is amazing and so helpful in getting through it. You can't do it on your own - at least I couldn't.

Chapter Six

We were now anxiously waiting for results from the MRI. This was going to tell us exactly how big it was, and possibly, if it went to my lymph nodes. We were going to get the results by Monday. Everything was such a waiting game. More sleepless nights ahead.

I do remember thinking that if anyone in our family had to get cancer, I was glad that it was me. If one of our girls had been diagnosed I think I would have immediately had a nervous breakdown. I had never been good under traumatic pressure. When Hannah was two years old, she almost lost her thumb. It had been accidentally caught in a door and it was dangling from her fragile finger by a thread. I frantically screamed "JOHN! JOHN!" He jumped in just as calmly as could be, picked up our daughter, and Ivy and me and drove us safely to the emergency room. I think I cried hysterically the whole way there. "She's going to lose her thumb! Oh my gosh, John! She's going to lose her thumb!" Needless to say, I didn't make anything better. Blood was streaming down her hand, she was crying and I was crying with her. I'm sure I scared our baby even more. John held it all together, as usual. He soothed our baby and me. And, yes, the doctors were able to save her thumb. I also would not have been able to handle it, if John were diagnosed with cancer. As I've stated a million times, he is my strength. I wouldn't be able to be strong for him like he has been for me. Without him I'm a little lost girl.

At this point I asked John if we could tell the girls. Our girls were headed to Uncle Mark (John's brother) and Aunt Teryle's house for the weekend to see their cousin Gabrielle. I heard through the grapevine that cousin Gabrielle overhead the news while listening to her Dad talking on the phone. Gabrielle said to her mother, "Hannah and Ivy's mom has breast cancer!!!" The last thing I needed was for our girls to find this out from a cousin and not from us. Especially, if they heard it and we weren't even there to explain anything or be there to comfort them.

John was going to do the talking. He was always better than me at keeping the conversation calm. I didn't have the grace that he held when it came to heavy matters. I was too emotional in that department and usually wound up crying. John always portrayed confidence and security, which was what our girls needed to see. He decided to keep it light. He called them into the family room and in a soothing tone he told them that mommy found something in her breast that she had to get taken out. And, that I might have some doctor's appointments in a little bit to get it out, but they were going to fix me up and I would be fine. When John had finished the girls looked at us blankly and said, "Can we go play Nintendo now?" So much for my theory that they needed to know. Off they went and I heard them start to play Nintendo.

Hannah did ask me a few minutes later, "Mommy, so if it was breast cancer and you had to remove a boob would you take off the left or right?" I told her I wanted to keep my own boobies. She asked another odd question that had the big "C word" in it. It is my belief that she was trying to decipher whether or not daddy was talking about Breast Cancer. He didn't actually say the word cancer. I figured her brain wasn't ready to process it. She would have come out and asked if she was ready. I was going to let it lie for the time being.

So that Friday night, our girls went off to Gabrielle's slumber b-day party. I had called Teryle in advance and she had Gabrielle sworn to secrecy, not to talk about anything. She had also explained it to her in a way that, I was just sick and the doctors were fixing me up. She commented to her mom "I knew she couldn't have breast cancer. Not their mom!" It's wonderful how children's minds work. They believe what they want to believe at times. I wish I could do this.

Every night I think I cried in John's arms. I cried and cried, "I just want this out of me!!! Get it out of me!!!!" I couldn't touch my left breast at that point, and neither could John. We both wanted this thing out of me!!!!!! "Why me???? Why me????" John tenderly consoled me every night. He swaddled his loving arms around me and told me I would be ok. I believed him every time. I trusted him to keep me safe.

This was about the time when we started seeking out doctor referrals from everyone we knew. Our neighbor Todd referred John to one doctor.

Our other neighbor, Janeen said, "Hands down, Dr. Zannis."

Gretchen's hubby John, an urologist, checked around and he said every doctor he asked said, "Dr. Zannis is the man." My ob/gyn also said Dr. Zannis was the best in town. We felt pretty confident we had found our doctor. My neighbor, Janeen, knew Dr. Zannis' wife. Janeen emailed her sometime that Saturday. She emailed back on Super Bowl Sunday with the kindest response. She told me not to worry, and that by no means, was this a death sentence any longer (which is exactly what I was thinking early on). She also gave me the number to the office and told me who to speak to, to make the appointment. After that, her husband, Dr. Zannis, also emailed my neighbor Janeen and gave me his cell phone number in case I needed to talk or had questions and to call him anytime.

I knew right then that Dr. Zannis was to be my doctor. "What a wonderful man! It was Super Bowl Sunday. What doctor gives his cell phone number to someone they don't even know and is not even their patient yet-ON SUPERBOWL SUNDAY? A good man! That is it who." It made me cry once more just how kind and caring people were.

Janeen came over in her jammies and robe to give me the email response from Dr. Zannis and his wife. We were all in our jammies too. Hannah had a good laugh at all of us in the hall in jammies and robes. Janeen pleaded for me to call him that day. "Call him RIGHT NOW or I will." I said I would.

She left and I realized I would feel kind of dumb. What was I going to say? "Hi there Dr. Zannis. I'm going to call your receptionist tomorrow to make an appointment with you." It was Super Bowl Sunday. I didn't want to bother the man.

Not forgetting my Facebook posting before I left for the party I entered:

Holly is WooHoo! Go Cards Go!

I wasn't feeling very WooHoo, but we went to Gretchen's Super Bowl party that afternoon anyway. I was taken aback once again by how nice people were to me. Gretchen and another woman Cherie had bought a necklace for me with the inscription "Believe". Gretchen I consider close. Cherie is more of an acquaintance and I thought it was so kind and considerate of her to even think of me. I had other people I didn't know well come up to me and hug me. They told me survivor stories of people they knew. I even had husbands coming up to me saying, "My wife told me and I'm so sorry. My mom had breast cancer too." To say I was touched is an understatement. We hung out, rooted for the Cardinals (our home team), had great food, drink and company.

The game ended, we lost, and Gretchen decided it was time to break out the champagne and do a toast. Not to the game or anything else, but to me. I just love her. Gosh, half of these people I didn't even know, and here they were lifting their glasses, toasting me. With my champagne flute in hand, I glanced around at all the faces surrounding me. Some looked at me sympathetically, some admiringly and lovingly, while others looked downright baffled and confused. And then I looked at Gretchen and we both realized that a big percentage of the people didn't know why they were toasting to me. It didn't matter. Gretchen said something funny, and everyone laughed. We then toasted. I cried, of course, but happy tears this time. Here I was again, being lifted up by all these wonderful people. Humanity is alive and flourishing here in Moon Valley, Arizona. People are beautiful. How lucky am I?

Before we left, Gretchen introduced me to Sharon. She

was a neighbor of Gretchen's and had recovered from breast cancer over a year ago. Dr. Zannis was her doctor. She was so cordial and told me her story, gave me her email and phone number and told me to call anytime. This was the first person, one-on-one, that I had spoken with who had recovered from breast cancer. It wasn't someone's mother, or my friend's sister or my friend's, friend's friend. She was right in front of me recounting her story to me. I remember her telling me that patience is one of the first things you will learn. Boy, was that the truth. It was all a waiting game. I expressed to her my surprise, in that I couldn't believe how much beauty I was seeing from something so awful. She told me "You will learn so many of life's lessons from this experience. It's an amazing journey." I promised myself at that moment that I was going to try to go through this with my eyes open.

I went home and jotted down on a scrap of paper:

> Believe. I do believe I will be ok. I believe even more that people are good; people are kind. I told my husband I always knew that people were nice. I just didn't know they would be so nice to me. People I didn't even know shared with me and wrapped their warm hugs around me to protect me. How lucky am I to be surrounded by such good people.

Not sure why, but I saved this. It is uplifting to me now.

(I know, I am a sappy person. It's sometimes quite embarrassing, but you are who you are. You have to keep in mind that I'm the type of person who will cry at the happy ending on Brady Bunch. Every warm fuzzy, every triumph of mine or someone else's affects me, and more often than not makes me cry. What can I do? I'm me.)

Monday came and I called Dr. Zannis' office for an appointment. We made an appointment for the following Monday. For a second opinion, I also made an appointment with another doctor, but my heart kept telling me Dr. Zannis was the man. Listening to my intuition and not wanting to waste the other doctor's time I canceled the second appointment. Being a strong believer in signs, I knew in the end I had to go with whom I felt best with and everything but the stars spelled Dr. Zannis.

That day I called my mom. I had finally worked up the courage to tell my family. I nervously dialed the number. She answered and excitedly told me that their friends from Australia were coming to visit. They were arriving that day and they were all heading up to the Grand Canyon and staying with them until Friday. I thought to myself "So, how could I tell them now? I wasn't going to ruin their vacation; much less someone else's who had traveled all the way from Australia, to find their hosts crying or upset the whole time. I had to wait a bit longer." Deep down relief swept over me.

Later that day, I had plans to have lunch in town with my sister-in-law Alisha, Stephen's wife, for her birthday. Alisha and Stephen had moved here a little over a year ago, to join the family business as well. I'm so glad they did. Not only are they great people and fun to be around, in addition Alisha had been very supportive to me. Her ears had always been open to listen to my tears. I know she has had to hear the same cries before, having dealt with cancer in her immediate family, so I was that much more grateful for her comfort. She is a wonderful person and I'm thankful to have her as a sister-in-law.

Before I left for lunch, my regular ob/gyn called. She apologized for not having been in the office for my initial visit, when I first discovered the lump, and she was so sorry to hear about everything. She told me, "If I had been in town, I would have just had you go straight into surgery and get it removed."

I instantly thought to myself, "What the hell kind of comment was that? Don't tell me "should have" at this point." I think I had asked her about the lymph nodes and she said you couldn't really tell until you get into surgery. We talked a little more about my recent experiences with doctors. Her friendly demeanor was always so refreshing. I hung up the phone feeling content. I hadn't realized though that our phone conversation was the discussion of my MRI results we had been waiting for. Had I been aware this was the big conversation, I would have asked more questions.

That morning, John was picking up all of the results from my MRI and all of the other reports for us to bring to Dr. Zannis. He drove the long distance there and then he called me perturbed that the doctor's office only gave him the MRI. No x-rays, no pathology-nothing else. You would think that since that is what they do for a living they would know what to include. I guess I had no right to complain about that, but come on, people. John told me that the MRI looked good. He read off a few details, but we didn't really know what we were reading.

I was in town now, so I told John that I would go to my ob/gyn and get copies of everything. When I first called their office, the receptionist sounded very annoyed with me. They told me I had to pay for copies. I didn't care what I had to pay; I just wanted copies. I had to have the papers to give to Dr. Zannis. "None of this paperwork crap was my mistake, so why were they treating me crappy. Hello? I just found out I have cancer. I wasn't asking for a sympathy song or anything, just the paperwork I needed."

Still in a good mood, I made it to the receptionist desk. I was going to overlook the phone call. Who knows what had happened in her day to make her crabby. Life wasn't going to stop around me since I had breast cancer. Again, the receptionist was really crotchety with me. I pretty much demanded my paperwork at that point, and one of the women finally retorted that she would make copies for me. I was hoping one of the doctors would explain the results to me as well. No luck with that. They called my name and I walked towards the open door. A receptionist stuck out a hand of papers and the door slammed shut. "Well at least I got the paperwork. Mission accomplished."

After leaving the doctor's office I immediately sat in

my car and started reading the report. "4.4 cm x 2.2 cm. Sounds big to me, but okay. A second mass under the nipple. Okay, I can deal with that. Everything good on the right side - No masses, lymph nodes fine. Okay. Sound goods." Then I read lymph node on left side looks worrisome for metastic disease. "What the hell is metastic disease? Crap! What about my lymph nodes? That was supposed to be bad if it spread to the lymph nodes. Crap! Okay. I'm not a doctor. I can't read this. I shouldn't even try."

Still feeling a little freaked out by what I read, I had something to drop off to Marv's office, John's dad. Marv owned many companies, Subway sandwich shops being one of them. This was the family business that John had joined a few years ago. He helped manage Marv's Subways. Marv also had allowed John to purchase one of his Subways. We were very thankful to Marv, since his generous act changed our entire life and our children's lives for the better. Once John joined the Subway team I no longer had to work. I had time for our children, for John and for myself. We were also very fortunate that we no longer had to struggle financially.

Knowing it would be rude, not to say hello while I was there, I popped in the office, even though I didn't feel like talking to anyone else that day. Not only was Marv there, but John's brothers Danny and Mark were there as well. They all asked questions. How was I? What the doctors had found out so far? Then they asked about the MRI. My voiced started to quiver. I started to explain and then I said, "You can't ask me these questions. I haven't had time to process it all yet." They all gave me the advice to call the doctor and have someone go over the results with me.

Every day I got more information and every day I had to process it all. It was all so overwhelming. More and more and more information! Each piece was so vital, yet I couldn't handle the intake. My brain would only allow me to process what I was able to handle. It's magical how our minds work. I would remember each piece just when I was emotionally ready for it and not a second earlier. Until then, my brain tucked it away from me, protecting me.

I left Marv's office and I think I cried my way home again. I'm pretty sure I started with the "Why me? Why me?" speech to myself again. I just wasn't strong enough for all of this. Plus, I hadn't had a good night's sleep in I don't know how long. I never functioned well off of little sleep. I called my neighbor Leslie. First I made sure carpool was set up for the day. I had been forgetting everything lately - kids included. Then I complained/cried about the report. "Metastic Disease? What the hell is that?" I hung up the phone puzzled, went inside and for the first time I logged onto the Internet. Up until that point, I had avoided it, because I didn't want to find myself searching to confirm anything negative. I was trying to stay positive. I had to know what metastic disease was though. Frantically I typed and up it popped. "Holy Crap!!! Cancer spreading. Crap! Worrisome for Metastic Disease. NO!! NO!!!!!!" I was starting to lose it. My wonderful hubby was still strong. Thank goodness for him. He again took over for me.

He called my ob/gyn, and left a message for someone to call back to go over the results. He called Dr. Zannis and left a message. He called his uncle, the radiologist, who was the first to go over everything with him. His uncle said it sounded like it was close to the chest wall and most likely I would be getting a mastectomy. Apparently, I had the better kind of cancer. I had invasive lobular cancer, pleomorphic type. He also said that more often than not, if you catch it fast, it doesn't go to the lymph nodes.

A bit later, my ob/gyn called. She apologized for not explaining anything in our conversation earlier that day. Before she told me anything and had me worrying needlessly, she had wanted to hear from Dr. Zannis. No need to scare me unnecessarily. (What did that mean?) She did prescribe me some Xanax so that I could sleep through the night.

Dr. Zannis called within the hour. He had John and me

both get on the speakerphone. I was thankful he did. First he explained that I didn't need to worry myself. He said this is all one day at a time. He told John and me that he was hesitant to go over the MRI report with me over the phone since there were many factors involved. "You have to look at the MRI, the ultrasound, an actual physical exam etc. and put all of the pieces of the puzzle together." He also said "You can't tell if it has spread until you get into surgery, so do not worry." He quelled all fears we had.

The next morning we were supposed to call his office and he would inform his staff to attempt to get us in even sooner. All day Tuesday he had surgery, but said if we could leave Wednesday open he would squeeze us in somehow. I think when I got off the phone with him I cried again. Happy tears again. What a wonderful man to call us at 9:00 at night, calm us down and then make a day of his hectic, to squeeze us in. Again, he had never met us. We definitely chose the right doctor. We also chose the right neighborhood. Caring and kind people surrounded us. I made a mental note to call and thank Gretchen again. I assumed she may have made her way over to his house and told him about me. Gretchen later told me, it might have been Sharon (how kind people are). That night I took my Xanax and slept like a little baby. I was ever so thankful for sleep.

Advice #10: Take some sort of anxiety medicine so you can sleep. You need your rest and the demons will try to rob you of this every night.

Chapter Seven

Tuesday February 3rd. That day I had an appointment with my primary care physician. To help speed things up, my ob/gyn suggested that I go do my pre-op approval and make my hematologist appointment. My blood disorder warranted blood thinners if I was having surgery. My primary care physician was booked so I saw another doctor in the office. She was a wonderful female doctor that made me top priority as soon as I gave her my prognosis. She did everything she could to help me; ordered all tests I needed, called Dr. Ondreyco (my hematologist) and made my appointment, and ordered test results from years ago from the heart hospital since I always had an abnormal EKG. She was so kind and constructive. I was so appreciative for this. Emotionally, I was going through so much every day that these little acts of kindness took so much pressure off of me. They also brought me a little smile. I felt confident that I was prepared. We were seeing Dr. Zannis tomorrow. I had my pre-op approval and my hematologist appointment. All was good.

Wednesday February 4th, 2009. It was my first appointment with Dr. Zannis. I was so anxious to hear what he was going to tell us. We arrived at Dr. Zannis' office, signed in and apprehensively sat in the waiting area. It was a beautiful office. I noticed the complementary colors of reds and yellows. Instantly I thought, "I bet his wife decorated this." It had a homey feel to it. It wasn't a stuffy or pompously decorated office. It wasn't a quickly decorated office. It was filled with love. I noticed the lamps, very decorative, with detailed paintings of tranquil birds flying about them. I noticed the rug, a beautiful oriental rug with apples blooming. I noticed the sofas, chairs and tables and how each thing complemented another. You could tell each piece was chosen very carefully, just as in your own home.

We were then called into Dr. Zannis' office. His nurse told us he would see us in his office first. We were directed into his office and we sat down. I again observed the décor. His office also had a very relaxing atmosphere. I noticed the awards on his desk. That was a good sign. Award plaques on the wall - voted best Dr. in Phoenix. That sounded good. He confidently walked in. We instantly felt at ease. He was just the nicest man ever. He gave us his introduction with background on himself and his practice and then we got to my chart. Calmly, he told us "This is no death sentence. You will meet some people that will have you in a coffin the instant you say you have breast cancer" (boy, was he right, myself included). He said, "Every cancer is different. Yours is different from your neighbors and different from her friend Suzie's and different from Sharon's." They were all different. He also told me to "Take this all one step at a time." This was the best advice anyone had given me to date, during all of it. These were actually the kindest words. He told me not to think about chemo yet, because I may not need it. Not to think about mastectomies, because I may not need them. It was all, one step at a time. Thank you Dr. Zannis for those words. They helped me so many times along the way, and when I didn't remember them, John did.

Dr. Zannis' Advice #11: Take it one step at a time.

We then followed him into a patient room. He asked me to change into the gown and said he would return. I quickly changed into a very unique patient gown. It was more like a shawl, rather than the customary cheesy paper patient gown. It was also pretty and dainty and surprisingly comfortable. I sat on the table and told John how much I liked the colors in the room; a deep robin's egg blue complemented by a sage green wall next to it. John admired the art deco style wood trashcan and medical cabinet. (Later, Janeen told me how much thought went into every single aspect of the office. Every last detail was carefully thought out. They wanted you to feel comfortable and loved - which you did.) I fiddled nervously and soon Dr. Zannis returned. He studied my films. He said he was happy that he didn't discuss the MRI results with us over the phone because he assumed I was coming in with a huge tumor. It wasn't. Yay! He did an exam on me and said that he didn't feel anything around the lymph nodes. Yay! He did say that you could never tell until you got into surgery. His expertise predicted that it looked like we could just do a lumpectomy since I had large breasts. He turned to me and asked, D's? I must have looked a little shocked. I replied with 38C. (Gosh, maybe I was a D. I don't think I want to be a D. I never thought I had such large breasts. I had actually always had a complex that I didn't have big perfect boobies. They weren't perfect, but apparently they were big. Funny.) He left the room and I changed back into my clothes and he returned.

We were told we couldn't make any decision until I had met with Dr. Ondreyco, my hematologist, to make sure my blood condition wasn't a factor in any of my treatment options. I was concerned that I couldn't take Tamoxifen, a hormone that treats breast cancer, because my blood condition prevented me from taking hormones. He said that maybe taking out my ovaries would be an option.

John asked, "Why not just cut them both off and give her new boobs so we don't have to worry anymore. Dr. Zannis explained that if we did a lumpectomy and then I take this tamoxifen drug for five years, my odds of getting breast cancer again, would go back down to any woman's risk walking down the street. Around ten percent. If I didn't get breast cancer, would I have cut off my breasts just in case I was in that ten percent?

"Hell no!"

He told us that I also needed to meet with a genealogist to do genetic testing. If I had the gene for breast cancer, then I would want to get double mastectomies and have my ovaries taken out. Having the breast cancer gene would bring my risk up to sixty percent to get it again, and again: attacking the left breast and then the right and back and forth. He told us he had great plastic surgeons that he worked with if I needed breast reconstruction.

"Oh my gosh! This is all too much information. Too much information!" I'm sure he told us more. (It's overwhelming just thinking about all of this again. Still too much information!)

He left us with this: "This is the time to get informed. You will be making some big decisions. Learn as much as you can so you can make the best decision for you. Ultimately, these are your decisions." We were advised to call once we had questions answered from Dr. Ondreyco. Dr. Zannis gave me a hug and told me to take care of myself. John and I left feeling really good about everything. This wasn't going to be so bad after all.

I went home and posted on Facebook a note with my encouraging news:

> Things are looking good – I saw the surgeon today.
>
> Wednesday, February 4, 2009 at 3:32pm|
>
> So I saw a wonderful, wonderful surgeon today. Not only is he a great surgeon but a great man. He reassured John and me that I do not have a death sentence. 90% of breast cancer patients survive - that's close to 100% in my book. As some of you know, I also have a minor blood clotting disorder so before we can set the surgery date I have to meet with my hematologist to get all that in order. I should know my surgery date by this coming Monday, which should be in 2-3 weeks. All looks well though. The doc did say that it is smaller than they thought - which is good.

(Thank you Shelley and Facebook.)

I also have to add it's ironic that such an ugly thing can bring out so much beauty. I can't even express to you how much warmth, compassion and goodness in humanity that I have seen in two weeks. Half of my tears shed have been over how nice people have been to me. I almost feel blessed to have this experience. (I said almost). Thank you for your thoughts and prayers. I feel I have this beat already.

Once again an outpouring of responses flowed in.

Vicki Way to take such a positive from this experience. Goodness in humanity can be so scarce these days; if anyone can inspire it, it's you!
So glad to know it's even smaller than they thought. And so you know, I've been feeling my boobies every other day since I learned about this.

Valerie Hey Holly,
That's great news! I'm really happy to hear that things are looking good. I've been thinking of you and John and the girls so much and am very happy to hear such a positive and encouraging update.
Sending you lots of love and warm wishes!

Alissa Hurrah, Holly! It sounds as though you have a surgeon who is compassionate and HUMAN....ahhh. I am glad you feel swaddled in love and warm wishes!

Gretchen Holly, so glad things went well with Dr. Zannis today. He's gonna take

91

good care of you!!! Love you, and thinking about you lots and lots! Love, gretch

Jeanne Great news! Thanks for keeping us posted! Warm fuzzies from us to you and the fam!

Cherie Hi Holly,
That's great news! I'm so happy that things went well. Take care and keep us posted.
Cherie

Kristine That is wonderful to hear. I have been wanting to call and see how you are doing but I have been afraid that you may not need any more interruptions. I just want you to know that you have been in my thoughts. Love you girl!

Janice Holly, such great news. It sounds like things are very good. We are sending good thoughts your way. We love ya --- you know.

Tammy Really wonderful news Holly! So so important too to have faith and comfort in your doctor-- Cheers to you and peace to you and your family! xox

People were so beautiful and so kind. I'm not sure I was deserving of their thoughtfulness, but I sure did appreciate them.

At some point I realized that life wasn't going to stop. It was all going to keep going. It wasn't going to stop for my family, not for my friends, not for our girls - not even for John. I decided I was going to keep going too. Whenever possible, I was going to keep life normal. If I could go to the girls' school, I was still going to go and help out. If I could drive, I was going to carpool and take the girls to all of their lessons. If I could work out, I was going to work out. If I could clean, I was going to clean. You name it. I wasn't going to stop living. Of course, there had been some days that I allowed myself to boo boo. I still had my boo-boo kitty from childhood that I had held on many occasions. I would pick myself up the next day after boo booing, and chug along. Everyone needs to pity themselves once in a while. I think it is somehow healthy as long as you have the ability to pick yourself up again quickly. I was one of the lucky ones, since it seemed to be easy for me to pick myself back up.

Friday February 6th, 2009. John had offered to go to my hematologist appointment with me, but I knew this one was no big deal so I said no. He called later anyway to see if I had changed my mind. Still I said no. I made my way to the other side of town and arrived early, so I popped into Borders bookstore. Taking Sharon's advice, I was going to buy myself a folder to keep my paperwork, reports, appointments, cards, pictures and any notes. I decided I was going to buy the most jubilant looking folder I could find. Not only was my folder helpful with relaying information to doctors, it was even more helpful emotionally. I included pictures of John and my babies and cards people sent me. Also included were all of my Facebook notes and responses. Everyone's responses were always so comforting. I felt like the guy in the cell phone commercial with the whole network behind him. At any given moment I had my whole Facebook support system/network with me everywhere I went. I was also able to lift myself up with my own encouraging words I wrote. When I wasn't feeling so strong, I could read my words when I was filled with strength. It would instantly pump me up with confidence again.

Advice #12: Take Sharon's advice and buy yourself a big happy folder and fill it with love (and all the other stuff you need).

While I was at the bookstore I talked with Julie on my

cell phone about how I was feeling. I was starting to feel a little bit guilty about being so selfish lately, but knew that was all I could do. "I just have to think about myself-at least in this stage. Hopefully, it gets easier." I told her how I was worried Katie would be upset that I didn't feel up to her party that evening. I just couldn't worry about her though right now. I had to focus on me and me alone. I know that sounded bad, but it was all I could do to get through the day.

I also told her about all of the responses I was getting to me having cancer. I thought she might have some insight, as she usually did. Most people I told I had cancer, would try to console me and such and would then switch to the problem that was at hand for them that week. When the first person did this, I was a bit confused.

I thought, "Wait. I just told you I have cancer and you are complaining about your busy day. Really? Busy day/Cancer? Really?" And then the next person did and the next person did and the next person did. They all did the exact same thing and complained to me. I wasn't upset by it. I was more curious as to the human nature behind it. Does it make them feel better? Are they trying to make me feel better somehow? Is it just fear? I hadn't figured it out yet. Julie thought it was because everyone I told loved me and it was hard to talk about. They had to switch conversations somehow.

Janeen later told me it was because they were comfortable with me and our conversations went on as usual. I was the only one thinking "CANCER, CANCER, CANCER." since it was inside me. They were thinking about me, but not nonstop like I was. They had their own problems as well. Life went on. All of their answers made sense.

A half and hour later I drove to Dr. Ondreyco's office, she had been my hematologist for years, and just so happened, she was an oncologist as well and worked with Dr. Zannis often. Good sign! I sat in the waiting room with other women that obviously had been going through chemo treatments, one with "the ugly hat" and another with very short hair. The one with short hair was super sassy and spunky. You could just tell she was gonna kick cancer's ass. She also annoyed me somehow. I think in reality I just didn't want that to be me later. "I don't want to have to be part of the cancer group. I don't want to be part of any of those supports groups. I DON'T WANT TO HAVE CANCER! I'm okay. Just one! Just one!"

They finally called me in and I had another long wait in the waiting room. It had been a few years since I had seen Dr. Ondreyco. My blood condition didn't require regular check-ups. I had a minor blood condition. This wasn't minor. She bopped into my patient room and I recognized her right away. She was short and peppy and very direct. "So, here we are, three years later." I think I asked her the questions Dr. Zannis wanted me to ask. I'm not sure. Again, it was all too much information. I did find out that my blood condition did not need to dictate my treatment in any way. After examining me she said my lymph nodes felt fine. She wished me good luck in surgery and off she went.

On the way home I made my few necessary calls. Normally, the first call I made I included all the details, every little thing they said and did. The caller would ask me questions. I would happily answer. I was optimistic. Things were great. I'll be great. I'll talk to you soon. Second call. A few details. I took a few questions. Things were great. I'll talk to you soon. Third call. Little details. I'm good. I gotta go. It was so draining to make call after call with so much information. Each time I would make the calls, I hadn't even processed of all the information myself. Everyone was waiting for results though. I shouldn't have even complained about that though. I'm grateful I had so many people that cared. It was just emotionally draining.

Advice # 14: Let other people make your calls for you or post mass emails.

I went home and told everyone I needed 15 minutes of peace. I sat outside by the pool in our comfy lounger trying to decompress all of the information I had received in the past week. I didn't want to think about doctors, tests, surgery . . . nothing. For just a moment I only wanted to soak in a little bit of life. I appreciated all of the flowers flaunting their beauty. I admired the proud trees standing tall before me. I soaked up the clouds bouncing around in the sky. Again, I asked myself what was the purpose of all of this? This time I was calm. I wasn't mad or frantic or petrified. I just wanted the answers. I drank in the beauty of our backyard and asked more questions. "What did God want of me?" I didn't have something huge in me. Maybe something little, but nothing huge to contribute to this world. I wasn't this shining beacon, maybe a little night-light, but definitely no beacon.

I looked across at the enormous tree in my neighbor's yard. Winter had seized its leaves. Soon they would be back but Mother Nature needed a little more time to nourish it with her warmth. The last bit of sunset shone its light on the edges of the tree. It was a beautiful sight. It was God shining. I don't know how to explain it. It just was. This made me think of my friend Julie. She always found the light of God somewhere, or at least she used to. She was a beacon of light, not me. I sure did miss that about her. (Her boyfriend is an atheist and now her light does not shine as brightly.) Maybe that was it. Maybe I was supposed to help her and then she could shine like before. Believe me, I know how that sounds, but it struck. Something struck me! I had to call her. Even though I was immersed, enjoying my moment of peace I had to. The last thing I wanted to do was get up and start the stupid calls again. I dreaded even looking at the phone. I had to though. Something told me I had to, so, I did. Julie answered and I immediately explained to her that I didn't want to talk, but had one thing I simply must tell her. I then rambled off the past fifteen minutes of thinking and my conclusion of how maybe that was it. Maybe God was calling her back through me. Maybe that was why God choose for me to go through this experience. She cursed me for telling her that. I said I was sorry for insinuating the blame of me getting cancer on her. That was not my intention. Something bigger than me moved me to call and tell her that though. (Again, I know how that sounds, but it just happened that way).

That Friday was one of our busier Friday nights. John and I were usually somewhat antisocial. We kept to ourselves more often than not, which was how we usually liked it. That Friday was different. John and the girls had plans for the Daddy Daughter Dance at 6:00, we had an engagement party to go to, hosted by Katie, a birthday party for one of John's friends, and the downtown Art walk where a friend's daughter was singing. I was excited for John and the girls for the Daddy Daughter Dance. After that I wasn't so sure. Sometimes it was easy to talk to everyone about what was going on and other times I just wanted to scream. "Stop it!!!!!! Leave me alone!!!!!" I just wanted to have fun like everyone else.

I thought and thought and I knew I wasn't really up for Katie's party. It was an engagement party for Krys, one of my close college friends. We still kept in touch but didn't see each other often. At that point she ran with a different group and had her own friends. Katie and Krys would be the only ones there I knew, along with our friend Anita, who rarely showed up for parties. Other than friends, Katie's family would be attending. I'd known her whole family forever. I felt certain I would have to answer questions about cancer to them and I wasn't feeling up to talking about it anymore. Maybe it was because it would remind me of my family. I still hadn't told them. (Tomorrow was the day I told myself).

I knew Katie would be upset, but again, I recognized I had to be selfish at that time. I had to do what was right for me. The idea was not so troubling any longer. Not saying I liked it. I just knew I had to get through it, however I could. So, if it meant hurting my friend's feelings and not going to her party, that was what I had to do. Sorry, Katie!!! I called Krys and Katie early in the day giving myself an out, just in case. Krys was cool, but then again we didn't hang out all the time. Katie said, "You won't have to talk about it. Just come for a little bit. It will be fun." As I explained, I wasn't up for it and how could I avoid discussing it with her family. That was impossible. My decision was made. I didn't like the idea that it probably hurt Katie's feelings, but I had to do whatever got me through each moment.

I wound up going early to the Zella Day concert (the daughter of our friend's friend) with Gretchen and her husband John. My John was going to meet us there. My John and her John always got along well and Gretchen never failed to make us laugh. They were good people and good times. We made it downtown and instantly I started to see all of these people from high school and all of John's high school friends. Everyone was aware what was going on since I had posted it on Facebook, so I ended up having to talk about it most of the night after all. An hour or two had passed and John showed up. He did the Daddy Daughter Dance then dropped the girls off at home with the babysitter. John was starved and so was I. I was starting to feel overwhelmed and was done with the whole social thing. I just wanted to go have a mellow dinner with my hubby. Gretchen and John were still into the concert so we went on our merry way.

We drove past Katie's (sorry Katie) and headed back to our side of town. Our wishy washy selves couldn't figure out any place to eat on the way. John kept bringing up the idea to go by his friend Shelton's birthday party. There would be tons of food and it was close to home, he pleaded. I really, really didn't want to go. Shelton was a great guy, but I didn't want to be forced to be social any longer much less be social with a crowd I didn't really know. John continued bringing it up and I felt compelled to comply. He had been catering to my every whim all this time. It was the least I could do for him. We stopped by for about an hour. We had some food, a couple of drinks, chatted with the few people I knew, and I tried to stay away from the ones I didn't. I wasn't in the mood to strike up new friendships. Finally, after about an hour, we wished

Shelton Happy Birthday and went on our way. I was happy to be home.

I had been on Facebook a great deal throughout everything. All of the positive responses truly did brighten my day. Each warm wish made me smile. Every smile was important in those days. When I couldn't grin, I would fake one. I knew that the muscles in your body, produced chemicals when you smiled that were sent to your brain signaling you to be happy. So I often mimicked the motions for a moment or two. Just doing that can make you laugh at yourself.

Shelley called me at some point and said "Oh my Gosh! We need to tell Oprah your story. The fact that we have been friends since 6th grade just makes it all the better. We talk every other week for years and have never once asked if we did our self checks." Now she sent me one posting on Facebook and I found breast cancer. We agreed, "What a great idea and we can be on OPRAH!!!!" Something good should come out of this.

Later I did get on Oprah's site and sure enough I saw on her hot topics "Are you too old to be on Facebook?" My topic was even better. Not only was I not too old, it (hopefully) saved my life.

I wrote out a five-page letter in the next day or two. I typed it onto Oprah's site and hit submit. "This will be great for sure." Red letters popped up PLEASE CONTAIN YOUR STORY TO 2000 SPACES. "Are they kidding? Two thousand spaces. I'm trying to tell my story of how I think I may be dying, and found out on Facebook, and trying to make it interesting enough so they will actually read it. How do you limit that to two thousand characters?"

I wound up with something like this:

I can't write this in 2000 spaces.

Facebook just saved my life.

Cut cut cut

Posting from friend

Cut cut cut

Found breast cancer

Condolences on Facebook

Cut cut cut

Very inspirational.

Oprah hasn't called yet.

Although, a week or two later I did see her hot topic was "How Facebook changed my life?"

When I saw that, I thought, "Oh, they saw my letter and now have a whole new topic for a show. She'll call for sure." I wrote another brief emotional letter, which I submitted on Oprah's website as well. She still didn't call. Maybe she was waiting for my book.

My oldest sister, Lorie, called me that day. She is a wonderful and intelligent woman. She also acquired my dad's hard work ethic, we all did, and his compassion. She had always been very supportive of me. She bailed me out on more than one occasion when I was younger. We have been very close on and off in our lives. Having my family living on the other side of town definitely distances me, though.

I couldn't keep this from my family forever. I figured it was time to tell them. Lorie was great. She was very encouraging and we found the humor in it somehow and laughed together. I asked her if she could tell mom and dad if she talked to them before me. Of course, she said yes.

I then called my sister Sheree. She is one year younger than Lorie, and a couple years older than I am. Sheree has always been the emotional one in our family. She had always been there for me as well. Sheree is a loving and compassionate woman. I remember when we were young, my sister, Lorie, was furious with me. Lorie had the evil temper in our family. After doing something silly to make her mad, she threatened that if I got out of the pool she would get me! I was around ten or so and I believed her. For hours I stayed in the pool. After shriveling up like a prune, I took refuge in our camper. My sister Sheree took pity on me and brought me lunch. I remained in the camper until my mom came home hours later. Another time, Lorie, mad again, tried to kick me but instead kicked the mattress. She broke her foot in the process. I thought she received justice. My parents thought differently. I wound up being the one in trouble for making her mad. I'm sure Sheree consoled me afterwards.

Not to say Lorie was always mad. We shared many nights giggling ourselves to sleep after sneaking into the kitchen with a handful of snacks. Sheree and I did as well. It didn't matter that I was three and four years younger than them. We were sisters and never failed to find laughter in something.

I knew Sheree was going to have a hard time hearing the news. She cried and cried, "You're my baby sister". It took a good fifteen minutes or so to calm her down.

"Sheree, I'm going to be okay." "Sheree, I'm not going to die." etc.

After I hung up the phone with her I called Lorie back and asked her to call Sheree and calm her down. We had another good laugh. I love both of my sisters. They are the best.

Two down, just my parents to go. I dreaded having to tell them I had cancer!

Advice #15: Get help from family in sharing the bad news with people.

Chapter Eight

I started thinking that I needed to take Dr. Zannis' advice and take this time to look at my options. John and I had the option to choose double mastectomies or keeping my breasts. Dr. Zannis was pushing for keeping the breasts, but he did say some people choose the other for sanity's sake. He also said, you can still get breast cancer even with a mastectomy. Since the implants are placed under the chest muscles with a mastectomy, the lump would appear on the outside of the muscle and would be detectable much sooner. I looked up on the Internet reconstructive breast surgery. There were a plethora of sites for plastic surgery. The breast implants looked great but what about reconstructive breasts. Then I found them. I wished I hadn't. Picture after picture depicted scarred breasts and none of them looked pleasing to the eye. Trying to be positive I kept scrolling, but I couldn't find any that didn't make me wince and instinctively turn my head to the side a touch. I switched to a different site. They were a little bit better, but not much. I wanted my boobies. I had never thought mine were all that great but compared to these I was "tits" so to speak. Turning the computer screen towards John, I scanned his face for his reaction and what I saw terrified me. The look on his face revealed that he was horrified as well. I think we then decided on a lumpectomy, if possible.

John's reaction to the reconstructed breasts had secretly scared me a bit. I started to think "Oh my gosh! In a few days I may wake up with one breast. I don't want one boob. I've seen after school specials about that with the woman standing in front of the mirror looking at her blank chest where her breast used to be. Oh my Gosh! Is that going to be me?" Then I started to think about John. "What if I do have one breast or really scarred breasts with tattooed nipples?" (That is what they do. If they cut off your breast they form nipples by tattooing the skin) "Will I be able to make love to him again? Will he be able to make love to me? He loves boobs. Will he still love me?"

That was a breakdown that called for Julie. Julie had been through all of John's and my hardships and triumphs. She was one person who knew how much John and I really loved each other. She knew each of us. John and I had our first vintage clothing store right next to Julie's vintage clothing store in Vegas. As you might guess, there were no stampedes to get into our stores and we had plenty of time to hang out on the porch waiting for a customer. We spent many hours in deep conversation. John and I have the fondest memories of Vegas and of Julie.

Julie had always been an advocate of our marriage. Her advice was never partial in my favor. It was always what was best for our marriage. If I had been unjust to John, she had no problem telling me. She helped me through all of our rough spots and I loved her for it and for many other reasons. Anyway, I called Julie and told her my fears. She reminded me how silly I was being. John loved me no matter what. He wouldn't care if I had big boobs or no boobs. He just loved me. I recalled the summer when John and I went to Alaska and worked at the fishing canneries. I had quit smoking, so to replace my oral fixation I ate all the yummy pastries they provided every two hours to keep us working twenty-four hours a day and I gained thirty pounds. John never once made a comment, never once looked at me differently. He was a great man. He didn't notice the outside, just me! And he loved me!

When I was pregnant with Hannah I also gained sixty plus pounds and John never made me feel fat. When I found out I was pregnant I weighed 114 pounds. I remember every month I had to make the long walk of shame to the scale at the doctor's office. Each month they told me that I had gained another ten pounds. On month five, they called me in to speak to a nutritionist. I was appalled. How dare them make me feel like a cow! I was pregnant. I really wasn't eating differently (except for the strawberry cream sodas I had every day). And I did quit smoking again, which I'm sure helped to slow my metabolism down, and I quit exercising. I was too tired to do aerobics any longer. The nurse warned me how she saw woman after woman become pregnant and gain excess pounds and then was never able to lose the weight. She scolded me to watch what I was eating and that I was gaining too much weight. I was livid. "How dare she!" At the same doctor's appointment I found out that I had a heart arrhythmia and they wanted me to wear a heart monitor for a week to check the status of each heart valve. I left the office in tears.

I jumped into my car crying and drove away eager to get to John. I pulled onto the freeway and immediately I saw the sirens flashing in my rear view mirror. Being pulled over by the cops was the topper for me that day. The cop walked up to me and sternly informed me he pulled me over for not wearing my seat belt. He inquired as to why I wasn't wearing it. I blurted out in tears "I just left the doctor's office and they told me something is wrong with my heart and I have to wear this stupid box to check my heart and . . . I'm pregnant and . . ." This is where the tears really come out "AND I GAINED ANOTHER TEN POUNDS!" By the end of my sentence I was sobbing. He looked at the heart monitor on my seat, my big fat belly (and most likely my double chin) and the tears running down my cheeks and told me to buckle up and head home.

Safely, I made it home, but the tears never ceased. I had gained thirty pounds and I still had four more months to go. I was exploding. I didn't want to be fat. (I had been chubby in high school and it was no fun. It really is true – people are not as nice to you when you are "heavy duty" as Ivy would say. I realized this after my first year in college. I came home for the summer thirty pounds lighter and everyone I knew before was much nicer to me, especially boys, or maybe I was just more confident – who knows.)

Walking into the store, I scanned all of the people, quickly looking for John. This was during the time we lived in the back of the store in San Diego. The moment I saw John I starting sobbing. His eyes widened, and he immediately asked me what was wrong. I was horrified. I couldn't even speak the words. He asked me again a little more frantically, "What is Wrong?" I still couldn't speak between the cries. He desperately pushed customers out of the store. He grabbed my hand and walked me back into our house (behind the back wall). Holding both hands, he calmly asked me once more, "What is wrong? Is the baby okay?" I could see fear building up in his eyes now. He was thinking that something dreadful was wrong with our baby or I had lost the baby. I had to tell him.

Breaking up every word with tears I spit out, "I . . .gained . . .another . . .ten pounds! I'M FAT."

"Oh honey. You're not fat. You're pregnant. You're supposed to gain weight." He held me close, as close as he could with my big fat belly. Thirty more pounds later for a total of sixty he still loved me, ever last chin and roll. He was wonderful.

And just to clarify to that nurse that destined me to be obese for life, I did lose the weight –HA!

The past month had been an emotional roller coaster for us, but we were trying our best to keep things as normal as possible for the girls. The girls had a sleepover at our house that night. We woke up the next morning and I took the girls and their friends on a long hike. It felt good to be in the open air. As I marched along up the mountain I couldn't help but think, "I'm in such good shape. How can I have cancer? How?" I was going to keep on hiking. Keep on living. I was going to hike this right out of me. Faster and faster I went.

I worked up courage all the next day. I'm not sure why, but I had been struggling to tell my parents. I love them very much, and I can't imagine how hard it must have been for them to hear that their child had cancer. I just knew it was going to be painful telling them. I also don't have the kind of relationship with my parents that we share everything, so talking about serious issues has always been difficult. Maybe that is what was hard for me - it was a reminder that I didn't have the perfect mother/daughter relationship or father/daughter relationship that you see in the movies. My parents weren't the first ones I called with good news. They weren't the first ones I called with bad news. Maybe that is what was hard. Maybe this was when I needed that wonderful relationship the most and it just wasn't there.

My parents were there for us girls in many other ways. My father as I've mentioned instilled our values and hard working ethic. My mother did what a mother was supposed to do; she cooked, cleaned, and drove us to practices. We never wanted for any necessity. When John and I first moved back to Phoenix, we lived with my parents until we found a house. I give my parents kudos for taking us in - all four of us. If you really needed help from them, they were always there. They were there to take you in, pick you up, fix the pipes, etc. I think this was how they showed their love. They grew up in a generation that didn't say the words I love you. It took some time for me to figure this out and accept. Not hearing I love you growing up always made me feel not loved. I think this is where my fear of falling in love originated.

I voiced this angrily to my parents one year during college. In tears, I cried out "YOU NEVER SAY I LOVE YOU. NEVER!" I can't remember all the words said, but I'll never forget that my dad came in my room later that evening and told me that his parents never told him either. He just didn't know how to express his love. He was never taught how. He apologized and I forgave him. I always remind myself that he was never taught how to say I love you. It's something I now teach my girls everyday.

While living with my parents I watched my mother give to everyone but herself, and it never brought her any happiness. I think it is because she never allowed herself anything. Watching her, I saw a bit of myself. I would forgo everything last little thing from the dress, to the lunch with my friends, to the lipstick . . . everything, so that John and the girls would have what they wanted. I realized it was actually selfish of me not to allow myself anything. I was causing resentment in our lives, not John. I vowed I did not want to be bitter about giving to those I loved. So I started something new in my life. Following Julie's advice I gave to myself. I allowed myself the dress or the purse or just a peaceful drive alone while John watched the girls without feeling guilty. I found balance.

Finally, I called, and my mom and dad answered on different phones at the same time. My dad, never one to talk about the important stuff with us girls, opted off the phone quickly so I could talk alone with my mom. Before I could say a word my mother said she was sorry about the news and sorry that I had to go through this. My sister Lorie had already called and broke the news to her. I was so grateful. She made it that much easier. I told my mom all the facts, assuring her I would be fine. I didn't want them to worry. We made plans for dinner with everyone for the next week and that was that. I did it. John and I spent the rest of the day with our girls. We were soaking up every minute with them.

February 9th. That day we had another appointment with Dr. Zannis. I was also stressing over some stupid Block Watch party my husband had planned for that evening. Here I was worrying if I was going to die or not, not to mention my new worry that I was going to have only one breast in a few days and I had to host a block watch party. I love my husband very much, but that was the stupidest thing ever - Completely asinine. If you haven't figured out, I'm a little bit of a perfectionist/OCD. I normally wouldn't have minded hosting a block watch party. With my personality though, that consisted of making sure my house was totally clean and putting out a nice spread. Especially if these were my neighbors whom I had never met before I wanted to make sure I made a good impression. Nothing wrong with that at all, right? Like I said, normally not a problem. I would have handled the stress, the cleaning, the shopping etc. But, things were not normal right then by any means.

Being the good sport I normally was, I wasn't going to complain about it to my husband. I was going to make the best of it. "Keeping busy would be good, right? Yesterday I had cleaned my home, so really, it was just food and a last minute tidy, and Oh, my doctor's appointment with Dr. Zannis." So, off we went to Costco.

I was thinking, "Okay, I can do this. I can host a party. I took my neighbor Leslie's suggestion and decided to make it easy and buy Costco's ready-made tacos and chimichangas, chips and salsa, and some guacamole; a little Mexican fiesta. I can do this." Leslie had offered to bring taquitos as well. I was in good shape.

We arrived at Costco and I hurried along with John following me with a cart. When I picked up the tacos he asked me, in his disapproving tone, "You're going to do those? There is something so much better than those."

I was thinking "Are you $#&*@% kidding me?" I tried to explain to him my dinner plan and what Leslie was bringing and that it would all be good. We kept going, I was putting more stuff in the cart and more criticisms came. "Was he serious???? Here I was trying to be a good sport about this whole stupid thing and not make him feel bad for planning some stupid #%#%$%& party on the day of my Doctor's appointment. I HAVE BREAST CANCER, HONEY!" Of course I didn't say any of this. I just turned down the coffee aisle and started to cry. "Just one! Just one!" Crying in the aisles of Costco was not my plan and quite humiliating.

He approached me and angrily said, "I'll handle the food."

Now my thought was "Oh No! He's going to put out some crappy lame spread and make me look bad."

I know I shouldn't have really been worried about what other people would think. When people enter a house though, it is a reflection of the wife, not so much the husband. The cleanliness, the style, what is offered, it is all a reflection of the wife, not the husband. I was completely stressed about the party, the food, my doctor's appointment, the possibility of one breast and so much more. We got to the checkout line and I was livid. He was putting things back, talking about putting out one subway platter, and to top it all off he was glaring at me. "He was mad at me!" That's when I lost it and went outside.

Frantically, I grabbed my phone and called the one person I knew would totally relate to this - Katie. I don't know how many times I said "Are you #%$^&@ kidding me? A block party? Tonight of all nights? Are you #%^$^&@%$ kidding me? I'm worrying whether I am going to have one breast in a couple of weeks. Are you $%^*!#% kidding me?"

I could always depend on Katie to agree and comment back "Are you &^$#& kidding me?" Thank you Katie for always being on my side.

John angrily loaded up the car and we took off. Our appointment was only an hour away. We both calmed down in the car. John apologized for the block party and told me not to worry about a thing. He was going to take care of it. I put my trust in him right after I explained the whole "it's a reflection of me" speech. I apologized as well. We stopped and had a quiet lunch. We got back in the car and were on our way to Dr. Zannis' office. We held hands tightly.

We were back at Dr. Zannis' office with good news from Dr. Ondreyco. I sat in the waiting room again admiring the loving décor. John was outside making calls to have our block party catered. Bless his heart. He hadn't realized the stress the party was causing me, until I blew up. He wasn't a wife. How could he know? He also didn't have cancer. His life was still moving; mine had stopped. John came back in and told me he was picking up platters from a Mexican restaurant right before the party. We both laughed and smiled at each other. Love is all forgiving on both sides.

We were called into the office once more. Dr. Zannis advised us to do a lumpectomy and we readily agreed without an ounce of hesitation. I asked him if there was any chance he would cut me open and realize that it was much worse than he thought and I would wake up with one breast. He comfortingly said "No, No." He told me that if he had to remove my breasts that would be a completely different surgery and he would call in the plastic surgeons to give me breasts at the same time. If I had a mastectomy I would walk out of the hospital with new breasts that day. No more worries. Yay! I was keeping my boobies. He also informed us that he was going to be removing two lymph nodes from underneath my arm, to make sure the cancer had not spread. We set the surgery date for February 24th and off I went. I always left his office feeling confident I was going to be okay. Life was good.

We rushed home and started to set up for the block watch party. The girls helped set up chairs and did last minute cleaning. John grabbed the food from a local Mexican restaurant and I touched up. Guests arrived, all women except for one husband. The food, I must admit, was delicious. It was so much better than the Costco fiesta I had planned. The policeman finished his hour speech. Afterwards, all the ladies stuck around and it wound up being ladies night out. A great fun filled evening.

The next evening I made my update on Facebook with all the new details.

14 DAYS AND COUNTING

Count down is on. February 24th. It's outpatient, which is good news. A little lumpectomy and a couple lymph nodes and I'm on my way. I get to keep my boobies!!! (I hadn't really thought of that part till a couple of days ago - Holy Crap, scary thought!) I'll be home by late afternoon. Then the next waiting game to see what the microscope shows and my genetic tests will come back 3 weeks later. If you're praying I don't mind asking to say a little prayer for me.

My Facebook friends impressed me again with encouraging notes and thoughtful prayers being sent my way.

Emily Good news, Holly! Stay strong and know that prayers are being said for you every night;)

Carol T-13 HOLLY....Should we get a little Dionne Warwick.. "Say a Little Prayer for You" going? XXOO Yeah Baby!!!!!

Tammy So happy to hear the news and also they scheduled it right away-- good!!!!!!!!!
Be thinking and praying for ya!!

Valerie Great! You'll be in my thoughts. I am coming to AZ at the end of March for a short weekend trip, so I hope I can see you then! Sending you all my love...xo!

Jeremy Holly, that is great to hear and yes you are in our thoughts and our prayers always!!!! Love ya~M

Vicki Yay, for you and your boobies. Now you can recover in the comfort of your own home. I'm thinkin' of ya lots!

Lisa great news....be thinking and praying for you.

Ruth Hey Hol,
Such good news! And of course I'm praying for you!

Holly Toner-Rose Hey Ladies, Thank You for all or your thoughtful comments and prayers. They truly help.

Jeanne We will keep the prayers goin' here at the our compound! Hope to see you soon! :)

Tuesday, I had plans with my sister-in-law Teryle, Mark's wife. She is just as sweet as can be. They live on the other side of town so we don't get to spend very much time together. She had called me at some point and told me she found a lump as well, and that her sister did also. I had described mine and told her that the chance of two sisters-in-law finding cancer within a week of each other was just plain impossible. The odds were so stacked in her favor. I told her I would go with her to her appointment in case her husband couldn't go. When I called her back, she told me not to worry that Mark was going with her and she would call me afterwards. I prayed for her. I wouldn't wish this on anyone.

It was time to tell the girls' school. This was really happening. It wasn't a dream. It wasn't going to go away. I had to face it all. I had breast cancer. First I called the principal and asked if she could set up a meeting with their teachers. I wasn't sure I could go through the painful task twice. Hannah's teacher called me soon after. I explained everything to her and asked if she could watch Hannah and let me know if anything changed: school, friends, attitude - anything. She wished me well. Ivy's teacher phoned next. Same routine. He was also very supportive. He asked who my doctor was. I said Dr. Zannis and he told me he had taught one of his kids years back. Good sign again.

Ivy had guitar that day as well. She took lessons from Ben, the same guy that had been teaching me the past year. I took a break from guitar during the summer time, so I would have more free time to just hang out with the girls. Since summer, I hadn't been able to fit it back in my schedule. I sat in the little waiting area during her lesson thinking, "Maybe I should tell him as well. I guess anyone dealing with our kids should know. Right? WRONG!" After Ivy's lesson, I asked him to come outside to talk while Ivy waited inside. Poor Ben. He was just a thirty-something guitar-playing hippy. He didn't know what to do with this information. As soon as I spit it out I knew I shouldn't have. His mouth hung open in shock. He stared at me like death was upon me. I then tried to make it better, which really just made it worse. So I tried to make that better explaining more and more, again making it worse. I finally stopped myself short, grabbed Ivy and ran to my car. "Oops!" I never brought it up again. The last time I saw him I was tempted to, but he looked like he was afraid to even look my way. I realized it was time to just Shut Up! That and I didn't have to tell everyone. Some people just didn't need to know. It's your choice who to tell and who not to tell.

That evening John and I also decided we would bring up the big "C word" to the girls. We had figured their teachers knew, all of their friends' parents knew, which meant some of their friends were going to know, which meant they would know. They needed to hear everything from us. John did the talking again. I was too emotional. John said we should keep it light. He was right. He calmly told the girls that what the doctor was going to take out of my breast was cancer. My little Ivy sat up and fear rang out, "IT'S THE CANCER!" She said it like, "IT'S THE MONSTER!" The boogey man had just become reality to her. My sweet little girl. And my poor little Hannah. As John talked she frantically organized her room. She wouldn't look at John; she wouldn't look at me. She just kept organizing, not even knowing what she was organizing. Afterwards, we did a little reading and said good night. Ivy was normal at that point. I think she forgot all about the monster. Out of sight, out of mind. Hannah, on the other hand would not look at me, would not give me a hug or a kiss. I don't think she knew what to do with her feelings. My initial reaction was to get mad at her, because right then I really needed to hug my little girl. I so regretted that I displayed any anger towards her. She wasn't able to process her own emotions yet. She was just scared and didn't want to deal with those frightful feelings. My poor little girl. I love her. I know her denial. Often, I've taken that same route.

The next day I wanted to make it to Hannah and Ivy's class. On most Wednesdays, I had lunch with them, and afterwards I would help out in Ivy's class, reading with kids. Ivy's teacher had assumed I wouldn't be there that day and had planned something else, so I went to Hannah's class to help. I was worried about Hannah after our conversation about the "big C." She wasn't talking about it, which meant she was worrying about it. Her class was still out on the playground for lunch recess. Off in the distance, I saw her pretty blonde hair flying around her on the swings. Her friends surrounded her. I walked to the other side of the playground where the swings were and said hello. Everyone said hello except for Hannah. While I waited patiently for her to warm up to me, I chatted with all of the girls.

She finally jumped off of the swings and flippantly said, "Don't you have a doctor's appointment to go to today or something?"

I told her I didn't until later and in fact when I saw the doctor the other day he told me, "You are going to be fine, just fine." She smiled and hugged me. She needed to hear reassuring words. She needed to hear that her mommy was going to be okay. All was well again with my little girl. I love her so.

Late that night, I called Teryle and found out that her lump was nothing. I was thrilled for her. I have to admit at the same time that a little part of me wanted someone to go through this with me. Not that I wanted someone else to get cancer. Heavens no! That was the last thing I ever wanted. I just wanted someone right next to me experiencing the same exact thing. I wanted to cry with someone, not to someone. I prayed to God to take those horrible thoughts away. Those thoughts were not what I wanted by any means. That might have been the night I first looked at the pamphlets and opened up the cancer book. I thought to myself I might have to join one of the support groups after all.

Advice#16: Support groups are there for a reason - support. Don't be afraid, like I was, to join one. (I wish I would have

114

sought out support for me and my entire family. My 20/20 hindsight.)

Chapter Nine

Wednesday, February 11th, 2009. So, it was my big genetic appointment day. I had my mother fill in the history on the medical forms the doctors requested, and fax them to me. There was no family history of cancer. I kind of knew what was going to happen at this appointment, so I told John I was good to go on my own. (Had I learned nothing from my first appointment?) They wanted to know if I had the gene for breast cancer. It was a two-hour appointment. What the hell they were going to do for two hours I wasn't sure, but okay. It was late in the afternoon and I showed up with book in hand, and checked in. I was the only one there. I could tell the office catered towards women. All the magazines were for women. The decorations, the frames on the wall, they all screamed women. Casually, I flipped through the magazines first. My mind was elsewhere. I glanced down at the table next to me. There, I saw the catalog of hats. Cautiously, I picked it up and slowly started turning pages. One page after another of really bad hats, next page - more bad hats, next page - worse hats. I abandoned the catalog instantly, throwing the poisonous catalog back on the table. I wasn't ready for that. Dr. Zannis' words rang in my head: "One step at a time." I picked my book back up and read.

Minutes later she called me in. She offered me a seat across from her desk. We each had a computer screen in front of us and she proceeded to give me a biology/chemistry lesson. She educated me on how normal healthy cells undergo changes over time and mutate becoming cancerous. She informed me of many of the possible factors that influence the mutation: a family history of breast cancer (which only accounts for ten percent of breast cancer patients), age, reproductive history, diet, etc. After her two hour lesson it came down to the fact that if I had the gene, my chances of getting breast cancer again along with ovarian cancer would go up to 60% or more. Then the lesson ended in, "Do you want the test to find out if you have the gene for breast cancer? It is $2000 and your insurance may or may not cover it."

"Was that really a question? I think the question is Can you come up with $2000 if your insurance doesn't cover it? Of course I want the test. Why didn't you ask me that two hours ago?" is what I was thinking.

She had me sign some papers and then she started to give me hotline numbers and titles of good books to read if you had cancer. That portion I appreciated. Then she handed me the "Ugly hat" catalog. This I did not appreciate. I wasn't ready for this. "Damn her! Why is she giving me this? I may not even need chemo." She must have sensed my distress and hastily started flipping through the catalog trying to find something fashionable I would like. "Let me tell you there is nothing fashionable in there. HAIR IS FASHIONABLE! I'M NOT READY FOR THIS!!!!!!!!!!!!!!!!!!!! Just one! Just one!" With hope ringing in my voice I asked if everyone loses their hair doing chemo and she said ninety-five percent do. That was pretty much everyone. I asked her if everyone had to do chemo.

Was there some chance in my dreamy denial world that Dr. Zannis would come out of surgery and say, "You are done!" Great Job! No more doctors for you. No chemo. You are totally done. No more cancer for you." He might as well top it off with a trip to Hawaii and scrap his office bill. She popped that bubble immediately.

She told me that because I was so young I was sure to do chemotherapy. The doctors were not going to take any chances with me. I was too young to get this in the first place, which was why I was at genetic testing. One bit of very useful advice she did give me, which I will give to you now. She told me to delegate. Delegate as much as you can and accept help. She said it is the hardest thing to do as a mother and wife but you have to delegate and accept help to get through this. I thanked her for the resources and asked when I would get the results. We were hoping to get them before surgery, since it would mean different surgeries altogether. She told me they were unlikely to come back in time, but with a little luck it might happen.

Advice #16: Take her advice and delegate. Accept all the help you can get. Accept the dinners, the cleaning, and the carpools. Every little bit makes a difference.

With little spirit left in me that day, I climbed back in my car, drove out of the parking garage and cried. I knew John needed a break from my tears and I had just called Katie yesterday with a "why me?" breakdown. I was trying to spread my tears around so no one would get tired of me crying to them. This time I called Julie and cried to her, "Damn it! It's not fair!! It's not fair!!!!" Julie asked me what happened that day. I told her "I got the ugly hat catalog. It's not fair!!! Why me????? This sucks!!!!!! This totally sucks!!!!!! CRAP!!! That's my word of the year. CRAP!!!!!!!! It's not fair!!" I told her how the doctor flipped through the ugly hat catalog trying to find something fashionable. How she showed me the fancy scarves. "SCARVES!!! I WANT MY HAIR!!! I DON'T WANT SCARVES!!! I DON'T WANT TO HAVE CANCER!!!!! I WANT THIS ALL TO BE OVER WITH!!!!! IT'S NOT FAIR!!!!!!!!!! DAMN IT!!!! IT'S NOT FAIR!!!!!!!!!!!! CRAP!!!!!!!!!!!!!!!!!!!!!!!"

It was a bittersweet day. That day John made his final payment on his Subway. It had been three-four years of payments. We were supposed to be celebrating that day. I felt like I had nothing to celebrate. Money just didn't matter.

All the way home I cried and cried. When I reached home John was already there. I tried to remain calm for him and hide my tears, but I just couldn't. It wasn't in me. I cried to him too, about the "Ugly hat" catalog. He, of course, was my rock once again. I tried on a few scarves and some hats and cried some more. Weeping, I whined, "I don't want to lose my hair." (Funny how you worry about your hair when it's really your life at stake.) We went to Target so the girls could get their school Valentines. I bought myself a big floppy black and white striped hat. I still didn't want to lose my hair, but just in case. Another Xanax and a little sleep.

Thursday February 12th, I had Hannah and Ivy's parent teacher conferences. Great news, as usual, from both teachers. We were very lucky. Our girls were such wonderful students. We were proud of both of them. I asked each teacher to please watch over our girls and watch for any changes. They both reassured me they would take good care of them and offered their sympathy.

During all of this, I went to the gym every day. I did my weights three times a week for thirty minutes, ran on the elliptical forty-five minutes three times a week and hiked for one and a half hours twice a week. Every time I ran I felt that I was fighting this. I ran harder and harder and hiked faster and faster. Damn it! I was going to beat this! Look at me! I was strong! I was stronger than cancer. I had beaten this already! I fought back the tears. I was going to beat this. I was.

One thing I must mention, although I have no idea if there is any connection at all. My doctors didn't know either, but who knows, maybe someone else's body has reacted like mine. About six months ago I started sweating much more than my body usually did. I noticed my body had a hard time adjusting to temperature changes. If I worked out I would sweat a ridiculous amount, then I would come home, take a hot shower, get ready and I would still be sweating a ridiculous amount. Before I left my house, I would wipe off the sweat and find that sweat was rolling down my back and stomach soon after. I was like the man in the movie "Broadcast News" who poured out sweat when he finally made it on the news as a broadcaster. That was me, and it was embarrassing. It was unusual for my body. Something was different. Looking back, that was the only thing that was different in my body in the past year.

Women kept saying, "You are peri-menopausal." I wasn't buying that. I was 39. There was something nagging at me telling me this wasn't normal. It will be interesting to see if, when I am cancer-free, my body stops sweating excessively. Maybe I'm wrong and I could be peri-menopausal, but something tells me I'm not. I hope so because I'm tired of wearing black. (It doesn't show the sweat). The only other thing that I can remember about my body changing is about one year ago a large amount of my hair was coming out in the shower for a week or two. Again, no idea if there is a connection.

Advice #17: Listen to your body. Changes in your body are your body trying to tell you something is wrong. Listen! (The sweating did stop.)

I made it to both of the girls' Valentines parties that day. I handed over my duties for both of the girls' classes as classroom liaison (someone's fancy name for class mom). My neighbor, Leslie, and I co-liaisoned Hannah's and her daughter Jessica's class so that was easy, and another mom took over Ivy's class. I wasn't sure what I had ahead of me at that point and I didn't want to neglect my responsibilities, so I bowed out. I still wanted to contribute and participate as much as I could. At this point, I felt normal and I wanted to keep things normal for our girls, so I went to the parties. They all had a ball. My sweet little Hannah in front of the class led them in the tooty tot (a silly dance that everyone had to follow step by step). She's my sunshine. And my sweet little Ivy too. We were so lucky to have them. God surely did bless us.

I was so happy that I was able to be with them: to help out at their school, to be there for the parties, to be a stay at home mom. It hadn't always been that way. When Ivy was three months old and Hannah a year and three months John and

I agreed that we hated Phoenix. We missed San Diego. We packed up our store once more and with Marv's help this time around we reopened a new store in San Diego. This was the biggest mistake in our life. We didn't realize what we were in for. I think we thought it was going to be like the first time around in San Diego. Happy carefree days. Those happy carefree days were gone. We had babies now, which along with happiness equaled stress. No longer were the days of bumbling down the boardwalk on our beach cruisers without a care in the world. We needed car seats and clothes and diapers and had schedules to follow and naps to take and more diapers. All of this meant we needed money and more money that we didn't have. So deeper and deeper we sunk and harder and harder we worked. I didn't have the time in San Diego to be the kind of mom that I wanted to be. John didn't have the time to be the kind of dad he wanted to be. We were too busy struggling to survive. We were thankful now that we had the time to be good parents to them, thankful that John had the financial means to support us without worries or stress, and thankful to be back in Phoenix with all of our family.

That night we had dinner with my family. I love my family dearly. I wish we were closer, but it is what it is, so I'm grateful for what we have. I always tell my sisters that we all turned out pretty good so we have no right to complain. Not everyone gets the whole cake. Sometimes you have to be happy for a little slice of it. I think our family has a little slice and that's good enough for me.

We waited for our table. No one talked about cancer. We discussed our girls, Lorie's son, Shane, who was away at wilderness camp, Sheree and Eric's daughter Gabby, and the weather, etc. I think my Dad probably warned us about the end of the world coming. (Hee Hee!) We were half way through dinner when my brother-in-law out of the blue asked me, "Are you on a diet?" My husband and I looked at each other confused. I wasn't fat by any means, nor had I lost a bunch of weight or gained a bunch of weight. Then I realized he was talking about a diet for treating cancer. There were things that were supposed to be helpful to eat and to avoid eating when fighting cancer.

I told him no and then I tried to make a joke out of it. I said, "What, I get breast cancer and now I'm getting fat too?" No one thought it was funny. I think my sister Sheree started to cry. So my usual self tried to make it better, and again I made it worse. My hubby, who possessed more finesse than myself, finally stopped me. I was never very good at my attempt at humor. One day I hope it will catch on, but until then I need to leave the jokes to John. The rest of the evening was pleasant. I reassured everyone I was going to be fine, not to worry and home sweet home we went.

February 14, 2009, Valentine's Day!! I leaned over first thing in the morning and asked John "Would you be my Valentine?

He leaned over and kissed me. "Of course." was his response. We had agreed a couple of days ago, with everything going on, not to buy each other gifts for Valentine's. We were so consumed with worry, who wanted to shop, or even had the time to shop? Both of us sat on Facebook that morning. I could see him on the couch with the laptop and I was at the computer desk in the kitchen. My thoughts kept turning to him.

John always made me happy. He is overflowing with charisma. He has something indescribable that radiates with absolutely no effort on his part and magnetizes you in his direction. His boyish charm, his witty humor, his good looks, his hearty chuckle, and his playful teasing, all make him absolutely irresistible. Women are attracted to him and men as well, not in the physical sense, but mentally. John has a way of making people feel good about themselves and people like to be near him. I've always felt so lucky that he chose me when he could have had anyone. I was the lucky one!

I thought back to the moment that I realized I was truly in love with him. Three months after John and I met, we planned our trip to Alaska. We were going to go work in the canneries in Alaska for the summer. This was a popular trip for many college students at the time. In fact, Katie did this the previous summer and had such a wonderful time that we followed her advice to go. We mapped out every stop on the way and every last expense. Realizing that we needed a big chunk of cash to get there we constructed a plan. I was going to live with my parents for a month and save up money and John was going to go to Las Vegas to work for Brandon and live with him and Brenda saving up money. After the month was up, I was going to drive to Vegas and pick him up, and then Alaska here we come! I drove John to the airport and dropped him off curbside and kissed him goodbye. As I drove away, looking at him in my rearview mirror, I heard a Wanda Jackson love song playing on my stereo. I was surprised by the emotion that stirred in me. Never had I had this feeling before. Tears started to stream out and I realized then and there that I loved this man. I couldn't bear to live without him. I was in love.

John told me I would fall in love with him and he was right. Months back while lying in each other's arms he sweetly said, "I like you, Holly."

I nonchalantly replied, "I like you too."

He then, a little more intently said, "No, I really like you." I was still afraid at this point of falling in love. Afraid of being hurt. Afraid of not being loved back. I didn't respond. He held me tight in his arms and knowingly chuckled, "You are going to fall in love with me." "Just you wait. You will." He was right. Three months later I was in love.

Now close to seventeen years later, we couldn't let the day go by without commemorating our love. It was Valentine's Day for heaven's sake! I sent him a private message on Facebook. I sent him the link of the band The Fleetwoods playing one of our unspoken love songs. Whenever we were feeling love for one another, I noticed a while back, one of us would start humming the chorus and the other would always chime in and finish the song. The next thing I heard was the sweet song starting to play on his laptop. He said, "I've always loved that song. How did you know?" My sweet Valentine. We kissed. I told him I thought it was one of our songs. (He didn't realize it and then I got my feelings hurt and then I apologized and so did he. Why do I ruin those moments? Can that please be one of my lessons learned through this????) After that, we decided we couldn't let Valentine's Day pass us by, without celebrating.

That night I prettied myself up. I slipped into my fancy, sexy low-cut dress. (Picture the famous Marilyn Monroe white dress, but black of course) This dress revealed some cleavage, which I didn't do very often, but figured I may not have the chance to reveal anything much longer, I might as well flaunt it now. I grabbed my wrap for warmth and off we went. (I never did take off the wrap that night. I couldn't flaunt anything. I realized the only person I wanted looking at my boobies was John.) We went to a local seafood restaurant. The restaurant had a band playing on the patio. We loved being entertained and what was better than some good blues?

Upon arriving at the restaurant we were told it was going to be a two and a half hour wait for a table inside. They offered us a patio table with no wait, but we could only order appetizers. Really, we had wanted to sit on the patio anyway, and appetizers were good, so we didn't mind. We sat backed up against the fence with all the tables in our view. Holding hands we watched the other young couples in love. Some looked excited, some bored and others downright mad. Lovingly, I looked at my hubby. I was so lucky. I had loved this man for seventeen years and he loved me. After looking around, I thought, "We look like the happiest couple here." The couple next to us took our picture for us. We laughed and talked and observed and laughed some more. The hostess called for the couple next to us and another couple sat down. We had them take our picture as well. We sat there for two hours enjoying each other. I think we had a total of four couples take our picture that night. Each shot got better and better. LOVE! We went home and cuddled up with our other loves - Our little girls. We snuggled with them on the couch and watched an old movie together. Life was still good.

That night I posted on Facebook:

Holly is love, love, love! Happy
Valentine's Day!

February 14 at 8:26pm

Advice #18: True love has brought me the ultimate happiness in life. I believe it is worth more than any riches in the world. I'm a true believer. Find your true love.

Chapter Ten

The next few days, worry pounded down upon me wave after wave. I started all over again "Why? Why me? Am I supposed to figure something out here? God doesn't want to take me. Okay. So I'm supposed to be a mom and wife and give back. Maybe there's more. Maybe I'm supposed to do something huge and make this big difference in the world. But wait, to do that takes tons of time. No, that's not it, then I couldn't be a good mom and wife. I'm too OCD/borderline ADD to accomplish that. I can only handle small bits and keep it all together. That's not it at all. Okay, so maybe I'm just supposed to make a small contribution in this world. Maybe I just have a little light to shine. Maybe it's my girls that will make the big difference. Maybe me being a good mom will help them do something to make a big difference."

What was it God needed me to figure out? "Okay, the girls and John. Life has gotten a little crazy. We've been watching more and more TV, going out with friends and leaving the girls at home, and spending more and more time on Facebook and less and less time with the girls. Maybe that was it. We needed to remember to stop and actually live. Okay, I can do that. I want to do that. I want to stop and live. I want to breathe in every moment we have with them. I want to breathe in every moment with John."

"And I want to give. I've been wanting to give. I'm going to give. I'm starting with my ten percent to some charity today. Maybe it's my little percentage and my little bits of time here and little bits of time there. Live and Give. LIVE AND GIVE! That's it!!!!!"

I said my "Our Fathers…." again and again. I found myself singing in my head "this little light of my Lord, I'm a gonna let it shine." Every night thereafter, I sung myself to sleep with this song. I didn't know why. This had never been a song I walked around singing. I didn't even know all the words, but it filled my head and my heart sang out.

Surgery was getting closer and closer, and fear was knocking louder and louder. No amount of exercise, no sunshine, no song . . . nothing would keep it away. I wasn't fretting about cancer or scars or hair loss. Now for some reason, I was worried I wouldn't wake up from surgery. My worry was that in a couple of days I would be dead. I'm not sure why I had such a fear, or where it originated, I just did. Graciously bowing down on my knees I prayed once more for God to spare my life. "Please God! Please spare me. Please don't take me from Hannah and Ivy and John. Please God! Please Jesus! Please Holy Mary! Please don't take me!" I begged God for my life. My body shook with emotion while tears rolled out then, (as they are now just thinking about it). I prayed and prayed 'til the girls came home from school.

I was feeling a bit overwhelmed. So many emotions were tumbling about in my mind. It was all so draining. I was on my way to the grocery store when John called and gave me the exciting news that our neighbor, Chip, had given him Phoenix Suns basketball tickets. He had three fifth row seats. Yay!!! Once back home from the store, John arrived home wearing a frown and informed me he felt like he was coming down with something, and for me to grab some girlfriends and go to the game without him. (I wonder if he really felt like he was coming down with something or if he was just trying to give me a fun girl's night out.) I thanked Chip and Janeen, and let them know that it was exactly what I had needed that day. Katie and my sister-in-law Carol came with me to the game. We had a ball. Someone brought up cancer and chemo and I changed my giggle to a growl and said, "I'm here to have fun and forget cancer. So let's have fun." And we did. We laughed and cheered and laughed some more. Girlfriends are a gift.

That night I lay in bed and prayed once more. That night was different though. First I said my "Our Fathers . . . " and then I found myself praying to Jesus. I had prayed to Jesus before in my life, when I was struggling, and found that Jesus carried me through those days. I recalled one minister's service (during our church shopping days). I remembered him preaching how in the Bible Jesus had carried someone through his struggles. You just had to ask and He was there. That night I asked. I prayed to Jesus for help, asking Him to carry me along through this. I vowed my faith in Jesus and in God. I was in His hands and trusting He would carry me through this. I prayed for faith.

Wednesday February 18th, 2009. I went to Hannah and Ivy's school to have lunch with them as usual. Ivy first, with her little gaggle of friends. I loved their stories, their chatter and their silly laugher. Ivy bounced off to recess and then Hannah came with her posse of friends. I loved them, too. Her group was a pool of smiles. They giggled for twenty minutes non-stop. I giggled with them. Off they went and I waited for Ivy and her class to return.

Ivy's class returned from recess and her teacher approached me and asked me if I could wait ten minutes to start reading. He informed me that one of the fourth grader's mothers was in a car accident yesterday and was killed. It was a one-car crash. She had just lost control of her car somehow and had not been wearing her seatbelt. The daughter Alana, was in the car as well. She was in the hospital recovering and she was going to be okay. The school provided a counselor on campus for the kids. Ivy's teacher and the principal were going to be having their discussion about the accident just then. Her teacher expressed to me how devastating this year had been. This was the third death this year at the girl's school. In the back of my mind I guiltily thought, "That's three. Bad things happen in threes. I'm going to be okay." I went outside to wait.

While I was waiting outside on the bench, my mind galloped with gloomy thoughts. "The poor little girl! Her mommy was her life! Her world!! I hope she has brothers or sisters. What about the father? Oh, the poor father as well! He just lost his wife." I fought back the tears. I selfishly thought about my family, too. This was my biggest fear for my daughters, and here this little girl, was having to go through that very experience. "She didn't get a chance to say goodbye. No chance to say, "I love you mommy." No chance for one more hug, one more kiss - Nothing!" I grieved for this little girl. (I still can't stop thinking about her.) She lost her whole world in one instant.

The classroom door opened and a little boy came out to read to me. Mournfully, he inquired, "How long is soon?"

I was confused by his question and with a puzzled look on my face I asked him, "What?"

He repeated himself, "How long is soon?" I asked him if he meant, was Alana returning to school soon, and he said, "Yes."

I explained to him that soon probably meant that she would be back at school next week. I told him that she was in the hospital recovering and when she returned home that her Grandparents would want to spend some time with her. Holding back tears of his own he quivered, "I want to spend time with my family." I asked him if he loved his family? He sang out, "I do. I love my family. I do." My heart poured out to this little boy, to all of these kids. They were all thinking of their families and their mommies. Death is so scary. It's not even your death that is so scary; it's the death that you leave behind. I thought even more about my little Ivy and Hannah. They were thinking about me, about cancer, about the possibility of me dying. I couldn't die! I couldn't leave them! Please God!

All day long, I thought about this little girl. When Hannah and Ivy returned home from school I asked them if they wanted to talk or had questions. I went over with them again the details of what was happening to me. My sweet Hannah confidently said, "I'm okay." She then explained to me that it's the word before cancer that is scary. She said, "If you had 'brain' cancer or 'bone' cancer that would be scary. But you have 'breast' cancer and that is much better. You can take that out." She was right, my smart little girl. It was much better.

That night I prayed for Alana and her family and her dear mother in heaven. I also couldn't help but think that God had just spared my life. I cried at the possibility that God took this little girl's mother in place of me. Just the day before, I had been praying for God to spare me. I didn't want another little girl to lose her mother. I didn't want it to be Ivy and Hannah who lost me. I didn't want anyone to lose. I mourned for her. I vowed to do something special for her. Something. What can make up for a mother missing though?

The next morning Hannah came into our room and crawled into bed snuggling close to me. She told me her tummy hurt and she wanted to stay at home. I told her she could stay with mommy and I held her tight. My sweet little girl, I know she started putting more and more pieces together, especially the news about Alana losing her mother. She was starting to think she could lose me. She couldn't tell me that but she didn't need to. That's what mommies do. They just know. (Don't take me from her God! I'm the only one who knows her just so!) We spent all morning cuddling on the couch watching Spongebob.

Later that afternoon, I had lunch plans with Gretchen. I wanted to be able to talk freely about cancer, so I asked Hannah if it would be okay if I left to have lunch with Gretchen. She was content to watch TV for a while. I kissed my sweet girl goodbye and told her I'd be back in a bit.

Gretchen and I had a wonderful lunch. We always did. We were both dramatic and sappy so it made for the perfect conversation. Neither one of us ever felt silly sharing our emotional thoughts to each other, since we both had them. I told her how I had prayed and then the tragic news concerning Alana's mother and how I felt God had decided to spare me. We both cried (in public). We usually did that too.

We discussed our team for the 3-day breast cancer walk. Katie had already signed us up as Team Holly Rose.

"Yay! I had my own team." We were planning on all kinds of fun fundraisers to raise our goal of $50,000. Our Team Holly T-shirt logo would be "LIVE & GIVE!" We laughed at my simple slogan. I told Gretchen how I had figured out what I was supposed to get out of this experience – to live and give. Never did I want to forget it, never take life for granted, and always remember my lessons learned. Gretchen and I finished our lunch. We talked more about life, not cancer, just life, our kids, and our husbands, etc. Life goes on.

I went back home to my baby, Hannah. We cuddled some more sharing stories and laughs, and Ivy came home a bit later and joined us. I love them so much. John came home and we all cuddled some more. They really are my reason for living.

That night during dinner we received a call from the genetic testing office. The tests had come back already. They asked if I could come in tomorrow to review the results. We weren't expecting the tests to come back before my surgery. I had been praying they would arrive in time, and they did. The results could mean entirely different surgeries. "This was good. Right?" I didn't think much about the genetic tests that night. My mind was still occupied with the fear that I wouldn't wake up from surgery. Mentally, I was at full capacity. I couldn't allow anything else in.

Friday February 20th, 2009. That morning I was ready to hear the news. I assumed that since the tests came back early, that most likely implied I did have the gene. That would mean I would be getting double mastectomies and my ovaries removed. I kept telling myself "This is good. I will know and not have to worry about it coming back. This is good. Right? I will just get new big boobies. They will be perky 'til I'm ninety. Good. Right? I will get my ovaries removed. I will just go through menopause early. This is good. Right?"

Before my appointment that afternoon, Margarita called me and announced that she had found a lump as well. Margarita, Marv's wife, is from Columbia. After thirteen years living in the United States she still has the cutest Columbian accent, sometimes indecipherable, but cute none-the-less. She wouldn't be Margarita without it. She is a good woman with a kind heart. Marv is a lucky man to have her. She asked me questions and I answered as best I could. I repeated to her what I told Teryle, that luck was on her side. There was no way two Rose women would find cancer in the same month. There was just no way. She informed me she was going to her appointment that week by herself. I advised her to take Marv or someone along with her, anyone.

After I hung up the phone with her, I called Brenda. We all called Brenda when there was a problem. I was concerned that Margarita wasn't going to tell Marv. Being from Columbia, I assumed it was part of her culture to keep it to herself and not cause her husband stress. I was also worried that if she went to the doctor's office by herself there would be the language barrier and she may not get all of the information she needed. I cried to Brenda. Here I was, still fearful for me and now I was fearful for Margarita. I didn't want Margarita to go through anything alone. John had been with me to every appointment. She needed her man with her as well. Brenda assured me she would call Margarita and for me not to give it any more attention. (Marv did accompany Margarita and she found out she had a benign lump that needed to be removed. All went well.)

I asked John to meet me for my doctor's appointment. Emotionally, I needed him for this one. We arranged to meet at Katie's house, since she lived down the street from the doctor's office. I pulled up to her house and my hubby was already there. He opened his car door and the first thing I saw was a huge bouquet of flowers in hand. He walked up to me and with a loving smile said, "I love you." I loved him too.

We drove over to the doctor's office. Once in the office, we sat down and she started going through her chemistry/biology lesson again and finally reached the fact that I did not have the one gene for breast cancer. Since they had not tested for the second gene she continued on with her lesson and when she was finished she asked if we wanted the second test. Again, was there even a question? The question was really, "Do you have another $650.00 for this one?" I'm thankful that we were fortunate enough to say yes. I'm not sure what people do who don't have insurance, or even have insurance, but still don't have money to pay their medical bills. We left, both feeling overly emotional. We had processed so much critical information that day, and every day before that for the past month.

Now I knew I wouldn't be forced to do the drastic surgeries. It was wonderful news. That would not have been good AT ALL. My mind was so not ready for any bad information earlier that day. I just kept telling myself that morning that it was a good thing. That way I didn't have to think about it too much. My brain was full. My emotions had topped out. I couldn't take any more of this. "I don't want this. Why me? Why me?"

John drove me back to Katie's and dropped me off with a kiss. I told him I'd meet him at home in a bit. Not wanting to miss Katie, I waited for her to come home to share the news. At that moment I wouldn't say I was happy or sad. I was drained. I was at the end. Katie walked up smiling. I told her the news and she cried for me. She cried happy tears. In the past couple of weeks I had cried so many tears. I just couldn't cry anymore. There was nothing left in me. I wanted this all to be over. Katie was so excited and happy for me that she cried some more for the both of us. I love her.

John and I had plans that night to have dinner with some friends. I really wasn't feeling up to it. Every moment I wanted to spend with John and the girls - no one else. I felt like I had to compromise though. John wanted to go and he had been through so much with me that I didn't want to disappoint him. So, the girls were going to their cousins and we went to our friends for dinner. The evening was very pleasant. We talked a little about what was going on and more just about life.

133

We were tired of talking about cancer and doctor appointments and cures. After a couple hours we said our thank yous and went on our way.

We went home, got cozy, and lit a fire. Lying in front of the fireplace, we both poured out our love for each other, our girls . . . our life. Gushing with admiration, John cried out to me, "None of it is worth anything without you. None of it." We both wept in each other's arms under the glow of the fire. He held me tighter than he has ever held me, and I held him back just as tight. I wasn't going to let go of him. I wasn't going to let go of our girls. I wasn't going to let go of life. I was going to live. I didn't want to die!!!

"Don't let me die!!! Please don't let me die, Lord!!!!! Please don't let me die, John!!!!" John told me I wasn't going to die. I believed him. I loved him. He made sweet, sweet love to me that night.

Our neighbors, Chip and Janeen came by the next morning. They were on their way to Guam and needed us to sign their wills. "Wills! Oh God! I may die! I need a will! What do I have? Everything I have is John and the girls. I should figure out special things to leave to our girls and to my friends." What did I have? My wedding ring, a few other pieces of jewelry I liked. I didn't know what else. What I had was John and Hannah and Ivy. That was what was important to me. "I want to Live! I want to Live and Give! Let me live God, please!!!!!!!!!!!!"

The next morning I realized that it was our last weekend before surgery. "I may not look like myself in a couple days. I may look deformed in a few days. John may not want me. I may not be desirable. I may look hideous." I called and reserved a room at a local resort thinking this might be our last chance for a romantic evening without me feeling self-conscience. It may never be the same again. We called and arranged for the girls to go to Marv and Margarita's for the night. Immediately after checking in, we went to the jacuzzi. We soaked up the serenity. It had been a month and a half of

134

hell. It felt good to at least pretend we were relaxed. We swam in the heated pool. John swirled me around and swooped me back into his arms. He wasn't letting me go. He loved me.

Back in the hotel room, I booked myself a massage. John drove me down to the spa and said he'd be back. After an hour massage my body still felt tense. I couldn't release any of my fears at that point. They were too close.

John and I had big plans for a fancy dinner and drinks afterwards. We decided on a cozy dinner and movies in bed. We were both aware that my body may not be the same in two days. I changed into my sexy lingerie. When I put it on, the thought came rushing at me that I may never wear something like this again in my life. I was mournful for me and mournful for John. We had a passionate night like never before and may never have again.

We returned home the following day and I now wanted my babies! I entered another post on Facebook:

> Holly Toner-Rose is missing her babies after two days of relaxation.

We were all having fun on Facebook.

> Brian Must be nice. I'll just stay home with Jock and eat dog foot.

> John Rose Gravy Train's the best (followed by Kibbles N' Bits).

> Brian Can you loan me some money so I can buy some generic dogfood?

> John Rose What happened to all that money you said you were makin'?

> Brian My wife is a slave to fashion. That's what happened to it.

> John Rose You say that like it's an excuse.

> Brian No excuse - straight up, balls to the wall, pedal to the metal, no holds barred,

reality (He said with a quiver lip trying to stifle a sob of anger).

<u>John Rose</u> Make a game out of it.

<u>Holly Toner-Rose</u> Hey Brian, will you ask Carol is she wants to go out to lunch tomorrow and do some shopping? Just some light sushi and a few tennis outfits. No big.

<u>Brian </u> Sure, I'll tell her as soon as she's done with her massage and pedicure.

<u>Holly   Toner-Rose</u>   Oh,   her   too. Sweeeeeeeet!

Facebook wasn't just a place to find comfort and encouragement, I found laughter, as well.

Advice #19: Jacuzzi, massage, relaxation and a little laughter.

Chapter Eleven

February 23, 2009, the day before my surgery. I'm not sure where my fear originated but I still couldn't help but worry that I wasn't going to wake up after surgery. My worries were compounded by other worries. I had convinced myself that if I could just train my brain in advance I'd be able to cheer myself on if I were dying, "Go back. Fight! Remember Hannah and Ivy! Remember John! Remember this little light of mine." I thought if I could do this in my unconscious state, I'd be able to walk away from the tempting bright lights of heaven. I reckoned I could cheat death somehow, if that was indeed my fate. I was going to keep 'this little light of mine' burning brightly. By being a good mother and wife and giving back I would shine my little light. I wanted my little light to shine some more. "Please God! Let me let it shine."

That morning I had a huge list to accomplish. I needed to do my final workout for weeks, shop for a present for Alana, go to Costco to stock up (who knew how long I would be down), and go to the grocery store as well. I also had lunch planned with Alisha and Brenda, I needed to stop by the girls school, do a last minute clean-up (again who knew how long it would be before I could clean again), find comfy surgery clothes, write my 'Just in Case Letters' (just in case), and go out to dinner, with John and the girls, with Katie.

I got a late start and figured one more day of not working out wasn't going to kill me at that point. I was already condemned to walking for weeks. What was one more day? Bound for Costco I went. I panicked the whole way there, calculating my time, to make sure I could fit everything in. I thought about Alana and started to fret that I wouldn't get everything done for her that I wanted to. She was my first priority.

After days of turning it over in my head, I decided on

giving Alana a basket of scrap booking stuff. My sister, Sheree, had done something similar for Hannah and she loved it. I wanted to present her with a way to help her remember her mommy. One of my biggest fears was that my daughters wouldn't even remember me if I died tomorrow. The biggest gift to me, as a mother, would be for them to remember me. I also figured if they remembered me, then they wouldn't miss me as much. Gosh, or would they miss me more?

Arriving at the craft store, I found a cart and searched for the happiest scrapbook I could find. I wished for Alana to be filled with joy somehow when she looked at it. I grabbed smiles and kisses and flowers and hearts. I grabbed bubbles and stars and letters and presents. My cart was stacked higher and higher. I grabbed everything I could to try to replace the loss in her life. What I really wanted was to give her back her mommy. I wanted my girls to have their mommy back again. I didn't want this little girl to go through this pain and I didn't want my girls to go through it either. Filling my basket with love for my girls, I was going to pass it on to Alana. My pretty paper and fancy scissors could never fill the void, but maybe they would give her a day of happiness, or just a little smile again.

My next stop was Costco. My mother nesting instinct was kicking in as well. I needed to make sure my family was taken care of. We were set for dinners. I couldn't believe we had two weeks worth of dinners planned for us. I had even turned people down. I was amazed by how giving people were. People we didn't even know were on the list to bring us meals. Ivy's class alone took five nights. Posts on Facebook came in offering to bring our family meals. Maybe this was why God allowed suffering. It brought out so much in humanity, so much beauty. I had seen more kindness and tenderness in the past month and a half than I had seen in my whole lifetime. Maybe God's plan was bigger than ours. He knew better. Maybe without death, we couldn't see life. I saw life. I didn't need to die. Others, around me saw it. I didn't need to die.

I met Alisha and Brenda for lunch (I loved that everyone kept taking me out to lunch). Brenda brought me the nicest gift. She had a bright bouquet of silk yellow tulips. She said, "These are very happy, like you, and will never die, like you." (They are still in my kitchen. They remind me every day to live and be happy.) We had a great lunch and everyone wished me well.

Not having the best handwriting, I asked Brenda if she could stay to help me write out notes for Alana's scrapbook. We came up with sentence stems to write in the scrapbook, for Alana to help remember things about her mother. We wrote, "My favorite memory with my mommy is...." "I loved when my mommy...." "My mommy and I laughed and laughed when...." "At Christmas my mom and I would...." etc. etc. Every stem we wrote I filled in with thoughts of my daughters and our memories. I couldn't stifle the tears. I didn't want to die. I didn't want my girls to be writing this out soon. I wanted to be here for them. I wanted to be with them.

"Please God!!!! Please God!!! I don't want to die!!!!" I prayed for myself and I prayed for Alana.

We finished just in time and I rushed it to the school office. I needed to bring it in that day because I didn't know how long I would be down after my surgery or . . . Tears started to flow again when I brought it in to the office. I was crying for her mother and myself, and her daughter and mine, all at the same time. I asked the office to give it to Alana or her grandparents when, and however the counselor felt it appropriate. Later, I heard that they had Ivy's whole class sign the card and give it to her. I was happy to hear that she liked it. I still wish I could give her back her mommy instead of memories.

After I left the school, I came home with the girls and did a "quicko cleano", and a last load of laundry. I relaxed for a bit and we all got ready to go to dinner. We had plans to go to dinner with Aunt KK (Katie). We met down the street for some sushi. John's brother Brian and his wife, Carol, came along as

139

well. As usual, we all had a nice time.

The girls always loved to see Katie. I'm sure I've said it before; she is like family. In fact, Katie was watching our girls the next day during my surgery. I knew she would make the girls laugh and keep their worries away, just like she did with me. During the past month Katie kept me laughing my fears away. Katie had offered to come to the hospital and wait with John during my surgery. I asked her if she could help with the girls instead. I really just wanted John there with me. John was the only person I wanted with me at that moment. It was the same when I gave birth to Hannah and Ivy. I only wanted John by my side. He was all I needed.

We finished dinner and confirmed all the plans for tomorrow with the girls. Katie had to leave and I gave her a card thanking her for all her help and friendship. We both hugged and cried. I told her I'd see her tomorrow and that I loved her. Brian and Carol wished me well for surgery and hugged me as well. I tried to be strong with them, but couldn't. I cried hugging them also. I'm sure Brian will be bitter with me for saying this, but I think I heard his voice quiver as well. (I've been so lucky to have such wonderful people around me through all of this. I feel loved by so many people. I don't think I appreciated this or really knew this before. Thank you everyone. I love you all, too.)

We came back home and I still had my last minute stuff to tend to. The next day we had to leave at 7:30 a.m., so I wouldn't have much time in the morning. I made sure I had a comfy outfit for tomorrow. I made my last phone calls to my mom and dad, my sisters, and a few friends. Then, the big one, I had to write out my "Just in Case" letters. I really was petrified that I was going to die right there in the hospital. I was afraid I was never going to wake up. The fact that I had never had surgery before, might have contributed to my fears. My only hospital experience was when I gave birth to our girls. Fearful, I sat in my bed with pen and pad in hand. I started with my letter to John. How to include in a few pages of notes of all of the wonderful feelings I had for him, what I wanted him to remember, about me, about us, our girls, our family, our life together . . . what I wanted to leave him with, how I felt about him, how I loved him, how we lived, no regrets, every bit of Love, Love, Love . . . HOW? I found no words could suffice. Nothing would be good enough. I didn't want to leave him. "Please God. Don't take me from him. He needs me. I need him! Please God! I love him!" I wrote what I could and hoped that he would know everything that I didn't write, through all our life, our love . . . he would know. I wanted him to be okay. (I love him so. I'm sobbing all over again just thinking back to it.)

I next wrote to our girls "Just in Case." Same thing. How was I to write in a few pages what I wanted to tell them throughout their life? I had so many lessons I wanted to teach them, so many things for which I just wanted to be there. I wanted to be there to tell them how special they were, encourage every talent, be there when they needed to cry and be there to cheer them on. "How could I do all that in a couple of pages?" They are ten and eleven. "Will they even remember me? Oh my gosh! I can't do this! I want to live! I'm going to live!!! That's it! I'm going to live! This little light of mine will not burn out tomorrow. I won't let it and I'm going to keep singing it and God won't let me die!"

Gretchen called me in the middle of this thought and she said, "See, if you're doing your letters that means you will be okay." I figured she was right. I thanked her for calling and told her John would call tomorrow with news. As I finished my letter, I sensed it really wasn't necessary. I was going to be okay. I could tell them everything myself. I completed my letter to the girls anyway, just in case. Knowing full well that I couldn't give them every bit of advice I would like to in a few pages I summed it up. I wish I could open it now, but I feel like it would be bad luck so I'll try to remember. I told each one how much I loved them and that I would always be in their hearts. I would always be with them. I told them to appreciate each other's differences. Sisters would always be there for each other. (I figured if I wasn't there for them, they could at least rely on each other. Not that they wouldn't have John, but he was a man. As a girl, sometimes you just need another girl to talk to.) And I told them something to the effect, that if I could pass something on to them, something I had learned in life, it was happiness. Find happiness. I told them mine was with John, and with them, our family. I found happiness in love, family, friendship, and kindness. Those were the true riches of life. I told them to search for their true happiness as well, (and to stay away from drugs). I found my babies in bed and hugged and kissed them goodnight. I told them how much I loved them just like I always did.

I humbly bowed down on my knees and prayed that night. I said my "Our Fathers . . . I prayed for faith that Jesus would carry me along through this and I sang "This Little Light of Mine". I fell asleep in John's arms.

Advice #20: Pray some more.

Chapter Twelve

February 24, 2009. That was the big day. It was coming out of me at last. We woke up early and quickly got ready. I was compelled to wake our girls out of their deep slumber, and adoringly hug and kiss them before we left. I went to make a last posting on Facebook and noticed there were already posts from friends on my page, wishing me well for my surgery.

> Tammy Thinking of you, sending good thoughts and wishes for tomorrow!

> Shelley Hey girl...thinking about you. Stay strong and try not to stress yourself out. Remember, the first few moments, what a great ride.

> Valerie Hey Holly... thinking of you and sending love and good thoughts, and will continue to do so, tomorrow and beyond! xxoo!

> Jennifer Good luck tomorrow Holly. Good healing thoughts coming to you from San Diego.

They brought me an instant sense of calmness. I made my post of Facebook before walking out the door.

> Holly Toner-Rose is feeling calm. (That's a good sign!!)

Immediately, wonderful postings with thoughts and prayers being sent my way appeared:

> Brian We're all thinking of you. You're in our prayers. Hang in there sister!

> Ruth I just got done praying for you

Holly!

<u>Valerie</u> Glad to hear it! You have quite a posse of loved ones out here all over place who are with you today in spirit.

<u>Alissa</u> Thinking of you Ms. Rose

<u>Emily</u> We're thinking of you!

It made me cry when John reread them all to me the next day. People were so beautiful and nice.

John drove me to the hospital. It was a good day. I could feel it. We checked in, and within minutes they called my name. John and I just had to answer a few questions and pay the bill. The receptionist asked John what check number and he said "444."

My eyes lit up as I said, "Oh my gosh. That's lucky, 444 right in a row. Good sign!"

A few minutes later the receptionist said "You know I'm not sure why, but whenever I see 11:11 on the clock, I make a wish."

My hairline must have moved as I shockingly replied, "Oh my gosh!!! So do I. I have extended it to 2:22 and 3:33 and 4:44, etc." "Another good sign!!!!! This is good."

We sat back in the waiting room. Another few minutes passed and they called me in again. They were quick there. This time I followed a nurse into a room. She was the kindest woman. They all were there. (I have to throw in praise for Phoenix Baptist Hospital. The nurses made all the difference. Thank you, ladies.) I changed into my surgery gown. Dr. Zannis entered, gave me his welcome hug, and went right to work injecting something into my breasts. I believe it was going to glorify the cancer in me. It would change colors or something to facilitate removing the cancer. I just knew it was going to help them get it out of me. From there, they wheeled me up to surgery. We grabbed John from the waiting room on the way.

They sent us into a small private room while we waited for the medicine to do its magic. The nurse gave me something to calm my nerves at that point, so that is where it all starts to get a little fuzzy. It didn't seem like we waited long. Soon the anesthesiologist came in. He introduced himself and John said, "Mr. Cypert, do you remember me? John Rose. I was your neighbor when I was a kid."

"Oh my gosh, another good sign. God was watching over me. This was good." Mr. Cypert sent me into Never Never Land. I told John that I loved him with a smile on my face, no worries - just smiles. He told me he loved me too.

They wheeled me away and I entered the bright surgery room and then . . . I woke up. Sleepily, I looked about me. I whispered, "I woke up." I heard the nurse comment something to me, and this time I chimed, "Yay, I woke up! I was worried I wouldn't wake up." The nurses all giggled. I think I giggled too. "Yay, I woke up. Thank you, God." I asked for John and within minutes he was by my side.

John was all I needed now. He safely brought me home and tucked me in. The minute I stepped into the door the phone started to ring. Katie was the first to call. I spoke with our girls for a minute so they could hear mommy's voice, giving them a sense of security, and I could hear their gleeful tone that assisted in repairing my wounds. My mom called next. Then Lisa showed up with flowers. Then more flowers came and more flowers came, even a basket of pineapple and strawberries shaped like flowers. "Oh my gosh! I felt so special!" I couldn't believe that all of these people were thinking of me. After that, it again got blurry. I slept and slept and slept.

John posted a message on my Facebook page when we returned home, so everyone would know I was okay. He posted:

<u>Holly Toner-Rose</u> is resting after a quick & simple surgery this afternoon. She's so

145

grateful for the support of her friends & family (especially her hubby).

Again warm wishes came posting up, one after another on my page.

Tera Hope you are doing well Holly! Let me know if you need anything =)

Julie That's great news!! I love you and I'm so happy to hear that you're doing well. Thanks so much for the note!!

Vicki So glad to hear you're done and especially that you've called the surgery "simple." This must mean you're feeling okay ;-)

Jeremy Hi holly glad to hear that all went well!! I look forward to the next update.~M

Dan Hi Holly im so happy you're doing well. I am returning to Phx Thursday. If you need anything please call.

Jeanne Rest away Holly! If you need anything, just holler!

Valerie Yay, glad to hear it, Holly! Keep us posted!

Brian John better be standing over you with a bunch of grapes and fanning you with a palm frond.

Karyn I am so happy it went well for you today. You've been in my thoughts and prayers.

Kristine Hey Holly, just wanted to let you know I was thinking about you. Glad to hear all went well.

The first day after surgery we decided to keep the girls at home. We thought it would be comforting for them to be near mommy. Even though I wasn't up and around they saw I was alive and I knew that would reassure them I was okay. I allowed them to play nurse to me all day. They were wonderful. I think I may have actually kept them home not for their benefit, but for mine. They were my laughter, my life, my healing . . . I loved them!!!

The doctor gave us instructions that I was supposed to remove my bandages the following day after surgery. There was still going to be tape over the stitches, but the big bandages needed to go. I asked John to help me do this. Walking into our bedroom I stood in front of my vanity and it hit me like a bolt of lighting. "I'm going to be scarred. Oh my Gosh!!" I hadn't thought of that really. I was so worried that I wasn't going to wake up. I wasn't thinking about my breast being scarred. "OH MY GOSH!!! I'm not ready for this." I told John I couldn't bare to look just yet. Lying on the bed I braced myself for some pain, physically and mentally. John gently peeled away, first from my armpit, where they took out the lymph nodes.

John winced and said, "That one is big. Ick!" He then started to peel back the bandages on my breast.

I held my breath. "Oh my gosh! Oh my gosh!"

John stated with a hint of surprise, "You can see the two holes where they injected you. They aren't that bad, Holly." Then in amazement he said, "Holly, your boob looks the same. It looks exactly the same. It's the same size, same shape, everything." I was so relieved. Gosh, cancer wasn't so bad after all. This hadn't been that bad.

Later that day I called Katie and Julie and proudly told them how great modern medicine was. "I don't even have a scar. Can you believe that? They just go through these tiny holes, chop it up with mini scissors and vacuum it out." (I've always been quite gullible). I told a few other people the same thing.

The next day I went to shower. I had John help me take off my shirt and sweats. Alone, I slowly took off my bra in front of the mirror. "Holy Moly, there is the scar! How could John not see that?" It was covered in tape still, but there was a scar. It went around my nipple from top to bottom. "How could he not see this? I can't look! I can't look! I'm not ready for this!!" I quickly jumped in the shower and tried to scrub the thoughts away.

I needed to start doing something to keep my spirits up. Depression was getting closer to my door and I had to keep him back. Exercise had always been my weapon of choice. A walk would be good, I decided. I slipped into my exercise shoes. That sure did feel good. It felt normal. I walked outside in the fresh breeze. February in Phoenix, Arizona was really spring. It was a beautiful day. I walked feeling strong mentally and physically. "One house, two houses, three houses . . . 10 houses. Oh my gosh! I'm gonna faint." Quickly, I turned around and went back home. I didn't have that much strength just yet. I'll go farther tomorrow I thought, back to the couch for now.

The next day came and I was still sitting and sulking on the couch. I was starting to go crazy. John and the girls were great. They waited on me hand and foot, kept the house clean, and life running smoothly. Dinners from friends and family came every day. I was so thankful for this. I didn't even have to arrange it. It was all done for me. Again, what a wonderful support system I had. I didn't deserve it all, but I was thankful for every gesture and every meal. I don't know what I would have done without everyone.

The next few days I didn't think about cancer. I didn't think I was cancer free. I didn't think I still had cancer. I just healed. My body healed, my mind healed, my family healed . . . Life was good.

Advice #21: Take time to heal.

Chapter Fourteen

Saturday, February 28th, 2009. I had been feeling so grateful for all of the wonderful people around me, supporting me, and my family. There were concerned phone calls and posts on Facebook every day.

Jerry Holly, how's everything? Hope you are doing well.

Tammy Hope you are doing well Holly!

Leslie Hi Holly, Glad things went smoothly! Time to catch up on all that day time television... that will get you back on your feet in no time! ha ha... If you need anything at all, just give me a ring!

Janeen Oh I am so happy to hear it was quick and simple!

Kate Hey Holly -
Hope you are feeling well enough to Facebook today!!

TonyaHi Holly! How are you doing? Been thinkin' boutcha!

Ruth Hi Holly! I've been thinking about you, wondering how everything went and how you're feeling??? LOL

Christopher smiles!

Everyone deserved a show of my appreciation, so I sent out another note on Facebook.

<u>Thank you everyone!</u>

I wanted to say a big thank you to everyone. All of your thoughts, prayers, flowers, cards, notes, fruit, (loved the fruit) the big basket of cheese, (you know I love cheese-hee hee) dinners, and every last kind word has been so wonderful. I can't even begin to tell you how special you all have made me feel. I think that is part of the fight and healing. Thank you again for everything.

As for surgery, all went well. Better than I had expected. I'm up and about moving slowing. We receive final news on Monday from the lab. I'm keeping my fingers crossed no wigs or ugly hats but who knows.

Thank you again for thinking of me. I'm thankful for all of you.

That was also the day of the Great Urban Race. I had signed John and me up for the event months ago. I had been so excited to participate in this. Obviously, I wasn't up for running any kind of race, so John flipped a coin with the girls. Hannah won the toss and became daddy's partner for the Great Urban Race. I tried my best to be happy for John and Hannah. I knew they would have fun. I even wanted them to have fun. Not so secretly, I was a little bitter about it though. I sent them off with a smile - I think. Immediately after they left I posted:

<u>Holly Toner-Rose</u> is trying really hard to be a good sport about not running the Great Urban Race today. (sniff sniff) Go (sniff) Team Rosebuds!! (sniff sniff).

A shower was in definite need again. Ivy helped me take my shirt off and I sent her out. I didn't want her to see the scar yet. I hadn't fully examined it myself at that point. I decided I could be brave and have a look. I winced at the thought. Looking at myself with my bra on you couldn't tell a thing. My boobs still looked the same size. They looked fine, totally normal. "Do I really want to look? Am I ready for this?" I took in a deep breath and slowly peeled my bra off. Surprised, I blurted out, "OH! It's really not that bad." The first look yesterday was very quick, which made it all appear much bigger. Another deep breath. Another look. "It really is not that bad. I can live with this. And maybe the cream Alisha brought me would really work and the scar would not be so dark. Maybe when the doctor took the tape off, it would look even better (or worse - don't think about that). I'm gonna be okay. I'm gonna be okay."

I showered and did my hair and make up, fabricating a sense of normalcy for a minute. Ivy and I then went for a short walk. Doing something in my usual routine and being out in the sun felt well. Exercising had always been a part of my daily schedule. Not to mention, it was my source of antidepressant, even in my normal state of mind. Now, incapable of engaging in any strenuous exercise, it was just one more thing I couldn't do. Happily, I did the only exercise I was able to do - walk. I must admit, I was proud of myself for forcing myself to get up and get out of the house for a short while. I hate to sound like I was tooting my own horn for these things, but sometimes it's the little steps that make a difference and only you can notice the little steps. The little pats of encouragement that I gave to myself helped me to take the next step.

Ivy and I returned home after our thirty-minute slow walk. I tried to keep going, picking up the house and going about my normal routine, but to no avail. A few minutes passed and I realized how exhausted I was, and how stupid it was of me to keep going. "I just had surgery four days ago. What was I thinking?" This sent me spiraling into tears. I just wanted everything to be normal again. "Like it's not bad enough that I have cancer, or hopefully had cancer, but I can't even pick up my house. I CAN'T do the Great Urban Race! I CAN'T go

151

out! I'm SICK of sitting on the couch! There are dust bunnies all over my house! IT'S NOT FAIR! Why me? Why me?"

After five to ten minutes of boo booing, I picked myself up, or I should say plopped myself down on the couch and cuddled up with the book I was reading. There was no need for me to wallow in self-pity. It really did no good. A bit later Ivy went off to her friend's house and then the phone rang. It was John calling on the road during the Great Urban Race asking for help solving a clue. I perked up thinking, "Okay. This can be fun. I can help solve clues via the phone. How fun! I don't need to be there. Fun, Fun, Fun!" Excited once again, I solved the clue puzzling them. I hung up feeling energized. A little bit later Katie called. I told her I had been boo booing since I had to forfeit my spot in the race. How, I was a little bitter about it, but trying my best to be a good sport, and feeling much better about it now that I was getting to participate via phone. We joked about it all. Then she told me, "I also just got a call from your hubby to help solve a clue." And she said, "Oh I gotta go. He's calling in now for help again." I hung up feeling deflated.

I angrily thought to myself, "Add insult to injury. Not only can I not go to the race, now you're going to take away my phone fun too. Come on! Where's the sympathy? I didn't mind one clue. I told them to call Katie if they needed help, but don't replace me. I want to have fun too. I signed us up for this!"

Immediately I called my hubby complaining. I know, not the smartest thing to do. He didn't deserve this. I really did want him to go have some fun, without any guilt hanging over him of me sitting at home. "And what did I do?" I called and chided, "Thanks for taking away my phone fun too!" He didn't hear me, so I had to repeat myself two more times. He still didn't hear me. Now I was regretting making him feel bad, so I had humbly changed my response to, "I was already sad that I couldn't go to the race and it hurt my feelings that you are not calling me for phone clues." He said he was sorry, of course. He further explained that they were searching for a clue near

Katie's house and Hannah assumed Katie would know the clue in her own neighborhood. Hannah was right.

I felt remorse for making him feel guilty, and still mad they replaced me. (Really, I was just upset that I was still stuck on the couch.) I decided I would not answer the phone and would forbid Katie to answer her phone either. Spiteful - just a little. Not one of my better traits.

I called Katie back and no answer. I left a message for her to call me back and joked about it. Katie was always able to cheer me up. I love her very much. We are very much alike. We can sarcastically joke to each other and we get it. That is what I did when she finally called me back (after she drove them around to clues - cheaters!). We joked about the situation. Complain/joke/complain/joke. I hurdled my resentment and told her she had my permission to help them if they called. I figured I could do the same had they graced me with another call (which they didn't).

After recovering from my self-pity and race drama, I picked up the computer and started writing, and writing and writing. A few hours later I received a call from John that they were on their way home. At this point, I was truly happy that they had fun together and without me. I didn't mind at all. Funny, how it all works out. In those few hours I discovered just how much I enjoyed writing. I think I found it very cathartic to tell my story. I may or may not tell it well, but I enjoyed it, so I kept writing. Anything was better than sitting in front of the TV, hour after hour.

I hadn't even found myself thinking about the possibility of cancer still in me, or new treatments to come. Maybe it was a sign that all was well or maybe my mind could only handle one experience at a time and my subconscious was aware of that, and protected me. That, or maybe it was the pain killers that kept kicking in. I do have to say that I tried to limit the pain killers. I had seen one too many interventions on people addicted to oxycodone after a surgery and their lives destroyed. I didn't need any of that.

That night I lay next to John. I was craving his tender touch. Surgery wasn't going to stop us from making love. I rolled across him, to the other side of the bed so I could lie on my good shoulder and we kissed. Then we made love and it was just as sweet as before. How lucky am I?

Sunday March 1st. The first thing I did was post my reminder to women to check for lumps on all of my friends' pages. I vowed after finding the lump in my breast, that I would send out a monthly posting on Facebook. Since, I found a lump I've had four women call me, telling me they have found lumps as well. All of them have been benign. Thank goodness.

I had been sitting on the couch all day since my walk, typing. It just kept pouring out of me. John was making fun of me hourly. He kept asking me if I was writing my Manifesto and threatening that he was going to buy me a beret. I have to admit that I had to ask him, "What is a Manifesto?"

He said, "That's even better. What color beret do you want red or black?" I didn't want a beret! I couldn't help but write though. It just kept coming.

Later in the afternoon I started to freak out. It was 5:00 and the house was still not clean. John went to yard sales in the morning and said he would clean when he came back. He didn't. Then he had lunch and told the girls to start cleaning and that he would jump in later. He didn't. He took a cozy nap and said he would clean after he woke up. He didn't. After he woke up, he got on the computer. This is about when I lost it. I nicely asked if he could help the girls clean when he was finished on the computer. I walked away looking at the mess around me. Okay. Granted it was not like a tornado struck our house, but as a mother, you make sure your family is fed and your house is clean. Since I couldn't do either of these things for the past week, for me to gain a sense of order I needed those things done. Meals were being brought in so I didn't have to worry about that. It was just the cleaning. My sister-in-law Brenda had offered to come over and clean my house for me,

154

which I had accepted. Brenda is the master cleaner. John, for whatever reason, declined her offer. He emailed her and told her not to come. I wanted to respect his wishes. Fine by me, as long as he and the girls wanted to clean. I simply wasn't able to clean and I couldn't deal with the anxiety of a messy house while being out of commission.

I strutted back in the office and asked a bit firmer this time. He had the audacity to look bothered, so I threw in the fact that he didn't let Brenda come. I know. I know. I should have just kept my mouth shut. But I couldn't. "Had Brenda come over, my house would have been spic and span. And she loves cleaning!" Now John was mad at me. I really didn't feel I should have had to ask in the first place.

He finally said, "Okay! Okay! I'll clean."

I walked back into his office apologized, and tried to explain to him a mother's need for cleanliness (or my OCD need). I wobbled my way back to the couch. A few minutes later nothing happened. I instantly thought, "Are you kidding me? He's in there cleaning his office." He was! This is when my tension exploded and I threw an even bigger fit. I stomped into his office and shouted out, "I don't care about your office! I could care less how messy it is for you to come sit and Facebook! I care what the rest of the house looks like! I care about the mess I see in front of me, as I'm forced to sit on the couch."

He grumbled, "It's not even that bad." So I marched room by room and pointed out what needed to be done. (What I normally did every week.)

"Could he not see the importance of this to me? This wasn't about him. It was about me!" I must announce that he did do a great job cleaning. After a few minutes of him cleaning, we both smiled at each other. I know sometimes I am out of control. I am happy that he puts up with me and my little fits. You also have to keep in mind the intense month we had just had.

The house was spic and span, just in time for another great magical meal. Not only did I not have to cook, I didn't even have to think about what to cook. It was great. Right around dinner time the doorbell would ring. In unison we all sang out "Ooooh! I wonder what is for dinner tonight?" This was something I would not allow John to veto.

Originally, he said, "This is too much. Tell people to stop sending food."

I sternly forbid it, "No way." In fact, I need to thank whomever it was who convinced me to say yes in the first place. It was so comforting not to have to worry about my family being fed. There was always a nice home cooked meal on the table. I'm so thankful to everyone. The meals were absolutely wonderful.

Tomorrow I was going to see Dr. Zannis with the results. "I feel really good. I think that is a good sign? Right? I'm ready for whatever is ahead of me. I don't care what it is as long as I am alive. At least that's what I am telling myself right now."

Chapter Fifteen

"So I think my book may be a little bit longer than I had originally planned. I saw Dr. Zannis today." On the way there I kept thinking "Good news! Good news!" 'til we were a mile away. Then the dreadful thought snuck in, "Oh Crap! I haven't been thinking I could get bad news. What if I do get bad news? I'm not prepared for this. Just one! Good news! Good news!"

We checked in and sunk into the super sofa in the waiting area. I read my book, and John read a magazine. They called my name and we were escorted to another pretty room. This time the walls were a dusty pink and a muted midnight blue. John delicately helped me undress and dress back into the sunflower/bumble bee shawl. As he did, he looked at me teasingly, sexily, and at both breasts. His playful look reassured me. He loved me and found me sexy no matter what - scar or no scar.

We waited a short while and Dr. Zannis came in. He got right to the point. "Good news and bad news." Good news was that he removed every bit of cancer out of my breast. I would not have to get a mastectomy. Bad news. It went into my lymph nodes. Dr. Zannis went on to say that he intended to take out two lymph nodes when, in fact, three were actually removed. One of the lymph nodes was full of cancer. The other two lymph nodes he had removed, cancer had just begun to seep into them. Now, Dr. Zannis had to bring me back on to the operating table to take out the surrounding lymph nodes, with the hope that the cancer hadn't spread further. He also informed us that I would indeed need chemo and radiation. This I knew anyway. I had been preparing myself for this unpleasant news ever since my appointment at the genetic clinic. I'm not sure if John was as prepared for this. Dr. Zannis informed us that the type of cancer I had was infiltrating lobular carcinoma, which was not an aggressive cancer. That was good. He didn't give us any odds. Before ending the appointment he looked intensely at John and said, "You do have to think about the possibility that she could die. She could die young." That was the part I didn't like to hear and John didn't like it either. I know he was just telling John and me, because he was required to, and yes, it was a possibility, but we really didn't want those ghastly words echoing in our heads. John helped me dress, and then he pulled me back and kissed me. John had to deal with thoughts of me dying. We scheduled the next surgery for the following Thursday. Oh, and more bad news I still couldn't wear deodorant yet. Later that day I posted on Facebook:

> Holly Toner-Rose is wishing her Dr. would let her wear deodorant again. P.U.!

Of course, there were responses to this one.

> Jeremy Oh no really-no deodorant?!?~M

> Ruth Deodorant? Who needs deodorant?

> Vicki Are you allowed to use "the rock"? It's some type of crystallized thing that takes away the stench but not the perspiration. Why aren't you allowed to use deodorant, by the way?

> John Rose The rock doesn't work (and neither does baby powder).

> Holly Toner-Rose It's just one side. Maybe if I just keep angling myself to the right no one will notice. What do you think?

After we left Dr. Zannis' office I started to go over all the up sides I could find. John stopped me and said, "I don't want to hear anything right now. I don't want to hear the good side. I don't want to hear anything. I just want to deal with the reality of it."

Once home I think I started with the bright side again,

158

trying to cheer myself up and cheer him up. He stopped me again and said, "Call me when you need me." I needed him a few minutes later. I only leaked out a few tears this time. Just processing tears. John went out for a bit and I made a few necessary calls.

"Good news/Bad news...." next call "Good news/Bad news . . . " With each call my nerves lessoned. I called Carol first since she had just left me a message. She had me laughing, of course. Katie next. Katie made me laugh, too. We laughed about the prospect of long spiral curl wigs, blonde wigs, wigs and boots. During my next surgery Katie was going to be out of town. She said she would send the flowers this time and someone could take her place. She said we'll just all switch jobs. I called Gretchen and she suggested we plan a day trip to L.A to shop for hats. We laughed and laughed at who knows what - ourselves. I called Leslie and we wound up laughing as well. It's a good thing for girlfriends. I called my family also. My sisters and I did the same, we laughed.

I posted on Facebook my Good news/Bad news note.

Good news!/Bad news

Good news - The doctor successfully removed everything from my breast!!! Yay!!
Bad news - It crept into my lymph nodes.
Good news - It only fully went to one. I'm scheduled to go back into surgery on the 12th to remove any surrounding lymph nodes.
Good news - It is not an aggressive cancer.
Good news - That will be the last surgery and the surgery is not too bad.
Bad news - Chemo and radiation. Kind of expected.
Good news - Fun with wigs!
Good news - I feel really good.

Good news - More time to Facebook.
Good news - I have you all to send me more happy wishes!!!
Good news - There's more good than bad news.

John returned home wanting to take me out for dinner. I wasn't really feeling up to it. I wanted to hang out with the girls at home, and we had a meal on the way, not to mention that I stunk. He went out for a bit alone. I enjoyed dinner with the girls and soon after he left, John returned back home to be with the family. I can only imagine what must have been going through his head. I had the unfortunate opportunity to think about my mortality throughout all of this. I think Dr Zannis' words struck him and he was now thinking about it as well. I wasn't going anywhere though.

As John was eating, I jumped back on Facebook to view the responses to my posting. I had eleven responses already. My goodness!! These always lifted my spirits. Each and every one of them was filled with inspiring and caring words. Humanity flourished on the pages of Facebook. More happy tears. Thank you everyone. This time I had John read all of the wonderful responses after he was finished with dinner. I think he needed some happy thoughts too and there was no shortage of them.

> Jerry You've got the perfect attitude. I know you've got this thing licked. You're in my prayers.

> Shelley I like your attitude! I'm not worried about you, you have a strong plan of attack.

> Valerie Yay for the good news of more good news than bad news! Thanks for keeping us all updated. You remain in my thoughts & prayers. axon!

> Jeanne Hooray for good news! You are

such a trooper! I am so happy to hear that you are in a great frame of mind! You are amazing! We are send many good vibes your way. We are here for anything you all need! Love to you and the fam!

Alisha___Holly, you are an inspiration. Truly attitude is everything. Go team, Holly! We love you!

Carol B Holly, I didn't like the bad news, but the good news is encouraging. Alisha got it right....you are truly an inspiration in more ways than one. There are a lot of people out here who love you. You are in our prayers day and night.

Leslie_ Yeah for the GOOD... I just have a good gut feel on this and know in my heart you are going to be fine! You have this thing beat, a good mental attitude is 95% of it! We love you!!

Ruth_ Good News - You can have a wig made out of your own hair...
Good News - Val's coming

Tammy_ I love your attitude and wish the best for you Holly!

Vicki_ Keep up the positive attitude. It's so wonderful. I think you are so awesome and are handling this like an old pro. I think of you and your family all the time and continue to send "good thoughts" your way.

Janice_ Hi Holly, Love all the good news and the good attitude. You are right, wigs are fun. We are here for you and whatever you might need. We heart you.

<u>Kate</u> Go Team Holly - And don't rule out the spiral perm wig. It was a really good look!
K

<u>Brenda</u>Holly,
We are glad to hear there's more good news than bad, but we want ALL the bad new to go away forever. You continue to be an absolute inspiration to us all! We hope you know without a doubt that we love you and that you are in our thoughts and prayers continually. I can't wait to come and do something to help you! Be thinking of something that's been bothering you around your house. You know how much I LOVE to clean and organize :) We'll talk soon.
Much love,
Brenda and family

<u>Jennifer</u> You'll be beautiful sportin' the wigs. Good news - your hair may grow back thicker. I am sorry that you're going through this and you're in my thoughts. Thanks for being such an inspiration.

<u>Margi</u> good news....MUCH more good news than bad! yay!

<u>Karyn</u> Always better when there is more good news than bad! Great attitude, it makes the world of difference, truly. More good news, it's only hair, it grows back. You have a lot to begin with, so you never know. Chrissy had chemo on and off for over six years and never lost all of her hair because she started off with so much. More good news, each time ... See More her hair grew back, it was prettier then

before. You don't have to limit yourself to fun with wigs; you can have lots of fun with scarves too! Love you!

Christopher Thinking of you often, and your attitude makes your body happy. Katie is right about the spiral thang! It worked for me. The angled look was a good one. I have pics to prove it.
xo

Holly Toner-Rose You all are so wonderful. I got on her to see if there were responses and OH My Gosh it just goes on and on. You all brightened my day!!! Big smiles and happy tears. Thank you so Much!!!!

Holly Toner-Rose OH, and I really did like your idea of the spiral perm Katie. I never got over them going out of style. I'm bringing back the big hair!

That evening, I was in Ivy's room helping her change her earrings. I looked over at her corkboard on the wall and noticed all of her notes from Santa Claus from the past couple of years, carefully tacked up. "You can't take me, God!!!!! Who is going to keep letters from Santa coming to Ivy? Who? Who will know when Hannah really just needs to get it all out, somehow? She's not mad. She's scared. No one else will know these things. No one else will go the extra mile doing those little things that only mommy can do. No one! Not even daddy. You can't take me. PLEASE!!!!!!!!!! I'm staying here.!!!!!! They need me!!!!!!!!!! I need them!!!!!!!!!!" I had to leave the room. I couldn't fight back these tears.

Again, I thought about Ivy and about Christmas and who would make sure it was special. My mind turned back to this past Christmas. We had set up the Christmas tree the night following Thanksgiving. This was always a special family treat. We would put on our Beach Boys Christmas music, all of

163

us singing along, while hanging the ornaments. Unwrapping each ornament was a gift in itself. They were little surprises, each and every one of them. Every member of the family had their own special collection to hang on the tree. We bought one or two new ones each year for each person, so by now we all had quite a few. I awoke the morning after decorating the tree, and there was Ivy in last years Christmas jammies sitting cross legged in front of the lit up tree. Her eyes sparkled. She was in an enchanting trance. Christmas was truly magical to Ivy. She believed in every last bit of it. So did I. Christmas was magical.

I heard Ivy's three year-old gruff voice in my head saying, "Merry Christmas Mom." After hearing it during the Christmas season she somehow equated it with the phrase I love you. So in May she was still saying, "Merry Christmas Mom. Merry Christmas Dad." meaning I love you.

Hannah on the other hand was our little detective. At age seven, while doing 'lay time,' she said, "This is veeery interesting Mommy. Look at Santa's note this year and take a look at Santa's note from last year. His handwriting got worse. It's almost as if a little kid wrote this one. Isn't that weird?" For years I had written the notes myself. Then, realizing Hannah would soon figure out that it was my handwriting, I wrote the note with my left hand instead of my right. I'm not sure what explanation I gave her, but whatever I said, it quelled her suspicions for a couple of years. Not taking any chances, the next few years I had my sister in charge of Santa's handwriting.

I also remembered Hannah's fifth Christmas. Every year on Christmas Eve we had my family over for Christmas dinner and we all exchanged presents. The girls were spoiled rotten by my family and received piles of pretty presents. The next morning Santa came to spoil them some more and the room was girly galore, filled with Barbies and princesses and Polly Pockets. It was another magical year.

That night as I lay with Hannah, I asked her about her favorite presents. Ivy was already fast asleep. I'm sure she was dreaming of herself in her new Belle costume riding on a purple reindeer to pick lollipops off the trees at Santa's workshop. Hannah went on to tell me her favorite presents. Then she stopped abruptly in mid sentence, looked at me confusingly and said "Mommy, where is my present from you?" She wasn't being greedy looking for another present, she just knew Mommy loved her best of all; so surely, I had to have gotten her a present. Somehow, in my eagerness to make sure Santa's arrival was unforgettable, I forgot to save and wrap anything from Mommy and Daddy.

My mind jumped to and fro searching for something to say. I desperately wanted to tell her right then and there, "I'm Santa, baby! Mommy bought all of that for you! Every last thing! Every carefully thought out gift. That wasn't Santa. That was Mommy! I do love you best of all!" I couldn't say that, of course. I remembered I had purchased a sweater for Hannah and Ivy, which I had forgotten to give them during the Christmas madness, so I ran to my room and came back with the sweater still in the plastic bag. She opened it up, not caring that it wasn't wrapped in pretty paper, and the biggest smile swept over her face. She wrapped her warm little arms around me and gave me the hugest hug and told me she loved it and she loved me. I hugged her just as hard as I could and told her I loved her too. I still wanted to say, "I'm Santa, honey" but I didn't need to.

I lay in bed that night and thought, "Wait! This all started with our anniversary, you know what number." A week after my next surgery was our 17th anniversary of the day John and I met. It was on the day after St. Patrick's Day. Maybe my doctor's appointment will be that day making it lucky. I can forget our anniversary year and start celebrating seventeen until January." I know that sounds ridiculous, but I liked it. (March 18th was indeed my next Dr's appointment.)

The next morning I woke up feeling refreshed. I was going to keep going. I checked Facebook and found Ruth's message. Ruth is an old friend from high school. We kept in touch every few years. She had always been so kind. She sent me a message asking me if it was okay to say, "That sucks." I loved her honesty.

"It did suck." I cried not because it sucked, but once again for how thankful I was for everyone. She asked if she could put me in touch with a friend who had just gone through breast cancer.

Since the beginning of this, everyone had generously offered support and said, "You can talk to my friend and this friend." I was trying to avoid that. I think I thought I could be strong enough on my own and I didn't want to bother people. After yesterday, I realized I was stronger with people. It was time to let the wall down. I requested to be her friend on Facebook. (Who knows, I will probably meet so many nice people joining the support groups. I really don't want to yet, but I'm going to start looking).

I felt good that day, almost normal, with the exception of my left arm. I went for a long walk marching to the singer Frank Black on my iPod. As I listened to the lyrics I thought to myself it was cancer that was going to lose, not me. I played it again and again and marched to the beat. Life was good.

After my walk I slowly undressed to shower. This was such a chore with my left arm out of commission, but I stunk. Carefully taking off my bra, I apprehensively looked again. Dr. Zannis had taken the tape off yesterday. "Gosh, it wasn't so bad. I can live with this. Just a tiny, moon sliver around my nipple. That's not bad at all!"

As I stood in the mirror blow-drying my hair, a task in itself, my positive spirit returned. I dressed in real clothes, (not my recovery sweats), put on my make-up. I looked and felt pretty. Everything was normal. "Damn it! It wasn't normal. Why me? Why did he have to say that? Why did he say I could die young? Why? Why? No! I'm not going to die young! I have two beautiful babies and John who love me. I'm not going to die! I'm going to fight this. I'm stronger than this. I fought quitting smoking and won. This was easier than quitting smoking. Hell, I've already won. I was crying in the closet day after day trying to quit smoking. I battled that for over a year and look at me now. This was so much easier than quitting smoking. I was addicted to smoking. I'm not addicted to cancer."

Yes, I smoked for fifteen years. I quit three years ago. Do I regret smoking? I don't know. You can't look back at your life and say I wish I did that, and I wish I did this. It is what it is. Could I have given myself cancer by smoking? Yes. Can I go back and change it? No. I'm not going to start beating myself up over could haves. We all make mistakes, just not the same ones. Smoking was one of mine.

I was smiling to myself in the kitchen reflecting upon my thoughts the past few minutes. I needed to write all of this down. This was good. This gave me confidence. "Gosh, maybe that was what I am supposed to do. Write all of this down. Maybe this is somehow my calling - to write a book. This could be an inspiration to someone else. I always wished I could be inspirational. I was hoping somehow, God would bless me later in life, with some beautiful harmonious voice, like Julie Andrews, to share with the world. Maybe He just didn't want it to be in song. Maybe it is writing. How funny is that? God hears. I'll take it."

Advice #22: Listen.

Chapter Sixteen

March 4th. Lucky day! Lucky Day! Dr. Ondreyco's office visit. I was unsure about what was going to happen today. I made myself a list to inquire about, so I wouldn't forget any of the millions of questions I had. My appointment went so much better than expected. Dr. Ondreyco slowly explained every last detail. Metaphorically, my cancer was like a dandelion. She said Dr. Zannis had plucked the dandelion out of me, but the tiny fuzzies could have fallen off the dandelion and could possibly be floating around me. Chemo was her almighty powerful weed killer and would blast all of the remaining fuzzies. If we waited, any one of those fuzzies could plant roots and grow more dandelions. She couldn't kill a bunch of new, fully grown dandelions with her weed killer, but she could kill all of the tiny fuzzies floating in me, if any. John initially seemed bothered by the thought of more cancer floating around me. I didn't mind since she had the weed killer ready and aiming.

She explained it all and outlined my whole plan with my prognosis at each phase of treatment. If I only opted for radiation my survival rate was only forty-one percent. I could add the drug Tamoxifen for five years and it would increase to fifty-nine percent. And if I choose to receive chemotherapy, eight rounds of chemo, each two weeks apart (that's four months), my chances of survival went up to eighty percent. One other IV injection, Zometa, could be administered once every six months for three years and would bring it up even further. Choosing all options, which of course I did, when all was said and done, I would have an 87% chance that it would never come back in my life. Add in my optimism, my wonderful support team, my faith and a little luck, and I was back up to 100%. We were even able to keep our vacation plans. We were just going to do chemo around it or in California if we had to. I had a few other tests to do: PET scan, heart test, etc. before starting chemo. I left her office this time feeling more confident than ever. She had answered all of our questions thoroughly. As we drove away, the material she gave us started to penetrate my mind and my spirit brightened. By the time we stopped for lunch, I was truly glowing.

"I'M GONNA LIVE!!!!! I'M GONNA LIVE!!!!!! I feel so good! I just know I'm gonna live! I'm gonna live to see my babies grow up! I'm going to see them get married! I'm gonna hold hands with John when we are eighty! I'm gonna hold my babies' babies! I'm gonna live!" (I'm laughing and crying and laughing and crying as I type.) "I'M GONNA LIVE!!! THANK YOU, GOD!!!!!! I want to climb to the top of Sunnyslope Mountain, and hold my arms high and shout out I'M GONNA LIVE!!!!!!!!!!! I feel like I did right after I married John. I can't stop smiling. I can't stop crying. I can't stop giggling. I've only felt this way twice in my life. I'm so happy! I'M GONNA LIVE!!!!!!!! God just gave me a voice!!!"

(I have to add that when Hannah and Ivy were born it was also a different kind of high on life. It was more of a miracle that I felt I was part of, and a peacefulness that swept over me. I don't want my girls to ever read this and wonder "what about us?" so I felt I needed to explain. I do that often.)

I went for a walk and proudly held my head high. God was going to allow me to live. With Frank Black blaring I marched on to the beat and the lyrics gave me strength to fight. I decided not to keep my ego. I was going to fight. Cancer was going to lose, not me. I marched on, noticing the hummingbirds, the flowers, the mountains, the beautiful sky and God. "You lose cancer! You lost the fight! I don't care about my breasts! I don't care about my hair! I don't care about scars! I don't care about you, cancer! I care about life! You lose, not me! I'm going to be okay. Thank you God!!!!"

I called my sister-in-law, Alisha, first. She had dealt with so much cancer in her family already. Her mother recently passed away from cancer. Her aunt, uncle, and grandfather all passed away from cancer as well. I wanted to give her some good news. She had been so wonderful to me and very supportive. I easily opened up to her each time she had called with painful tears. I wanted to give her happy tears.

I called Julie. We cried, more happy tears. I also told her, that I wished that she had God in her life more again. I had missed our talks. Neither one of us went to church, but we fully believed. We had a stronger faith than some sitting in their churches. Somewhere along the line we just stopped talking about God. I think that is why God wants you to go to church. It helps to keep your faith strong. Our friendship and talks were church to us, but that was lost. I wanted that back. I missed that with her.

I called Katie, We hollered, "YAY!!!" And hollered some more. "YAY!!! I was gonna live!!!!!!!!"

John's brother Danny called me to see how I was doing. Danny also wanted to know how John was holding up. He told me how John was distraught a few days ago (after our last visit with Dr. Zannis). I was secretly a little happy to hear that John was upset. I hadn't seen any tears except for our one emotional night in front of the fireplace. Every day he had been strong for me. I didn't even have to dig deep for that. I just knew he was strong. Somehow, though, the confirmation of his concern was a confirmation of our love as well. Not that I wanted him to worry or to be crying every day like me. I guess it's just human nature to want the person you love to worry about you. Stupid, I know. I love him so and am so happy he loves me.

The girls came home and I told them the good news as well. Mommy was going to live! I was going to be there every moment with them.

We went out to celebrate with Katie for dinner.

I was so excited once again, that I had to post something on Facebook. I was sure people were getting tired of my notes and postings, but I wanted to share my wonderful news. All of these people were thinking of me, supporting me. I wanted to present them good news!! The next morning I posted another note.

GOOD NEWS! GOOD NEWS! GOOD NEWS!

So I hate to bombard you all with another note but I'm just so happy I wanted to share my good news with all of you. I went to my oncologist yesterday and she went over the whole plan with John and me. After chemo, radiation and some other drugs when all is said and done I'm at an 87% survival rate that this will never come back again in my lifetime. Throw in my optimism, my wonderful support system, my faith and a little bit of luck and I'm back up to 100%. Yay!!!!!! I'm gonna live. I just know it. I'm gonna see my babies have babies and hold hands with my hubby when I'm 80. Thank you everyone for all your wonderful prayers. God was listening. I'm going to be o.k. Thank you for listening to me as well. You have been just wonderful. Gosh, I just thought Facebook was a great way to procrastinate. Who knew it would be an added support system! THANK YOU!!!!!!!!!!!

I felt like I had the whole world cheering me on.

<u>Margi</u> This is GREAT news Holly! SO happy for you and John!!!

<u>Jerry</u> Wonderful!!! I'm very happy for you.

<u>Valerie</u> Yay!!!! Great news indeed! So happy to hear it!

<u>Lorraine</u> Glad to hear the news!!! God is good. Those prayer chains work wonders.

:) I love you, sis.

Kristine That is wonderful news Holly!

Tammy Such amazing news Holly! You make all this happen!

Anna GO HOLLY!!

Tonya Awesome! You are an amazing woman and an inspiration. Your optimism throughout everything has been incredible!

Jeremy Holly, words cannot express just how happy I am for you and your family!!! All my love to you and yours holly. Love you~M

Christopher Wonderful news - power of positive thinking
xo
C

Emily Great news, Holly! Hooray!

Ruth Woo hoo! Now you just need to continue to find humorous things every day because laughter is healing... we'll all be healthier by laughing with you! :o)

Jeanne Awesome news! Way to fight!

Janice yeah!!!!!!!!!

Stacie Awesome news...you are loved! ;)

Teri That's wonderful news Holly! You're going to beat this thing! Hope to see you soon!

Dawn Please...you are going to make it...you will have many years of hearing me whine about the Navy.... you aren't getting off that easy! Anyway..love you and very happy to hear the good news! Cancer Smancer...you will kick it in its ass!

H. Shelton Amen. The Valentine clan is very happy for you. Thanks for the update.

Matt Everyone in Ohio is VERY HAPPY for you and your family! Great news cuz!

Karyn Never a doubt!

Brandon Holly, so now that that's over, what else do you want to do!? HAHA! So great to hear the good news Holly. You're always in our thoughts and prayers, you know.

Shelley I couldn't be happier for you! You are a great example for everyone!

Leslie You ROCK Holly!! Great news!

Jennifer Yay Yay Yay!

Vicki Fantastic! Your updates are so awesome to read. If this were wrestling, you'd have this thing "pinned."

Carol Well, Holly if good cheer counts for anything, (and it does.. because I played a doctor on TV) you got this thing licked. XXOO

Gretchen Holly, you know we love you!!!!!!!

I was completely amazed by how incredibly blessed I was to have so many wonderful people on my side cheering me on and cheering me up.

I then posted:

Holly Toner-Rose is happy!!!!!!!!

173

Thirty Minutes later. OH MY GOSH!!! OPRAH JUST CALLED!!!!!! Okay, so not Oprah, but someone from the Oprah show!!!!! I was talking to Gretchen on the phone when she beeped in. She introduced herself as Megan . . . and asked if I could talk. "HELLO, IT WAS THE OPRAH SHOW! Of course, I could talk!" She asked me how long I had been on Facebook. I told her that it was my husband who first joined. Watching him every night on Facebook, I felt I was missing out on all the fun, so I joined as well a few months back. She asked if I enjoyed it. I told her yes and how I talked to friends new and old, and how I met up with Vicki and was now hiking with her every week. She asked about the posting I received on Facebook and I explained what it was, and how Shelley had sent it to me, and consequently, I found a lump upon doing my self-check. She then asked me to tell my story.

"Oh my gosh! So much has happened in the past month and half. What do I say now?" was running through my head. I started at the beginning. At some point I started to cry. I think I may have had her crying too, so I stopped and said, "Wait, the ending is happy!" I kept on with my story. She stopped me at some point and said she was being called into a meeting. She asked if she could give me an email and if I could send some pictures. I asked if I could friend her on Facebook instead. Then, she asked if she could call back and I said "No, I was going to meet my sisters-in-law for lunch." (Who tells Oprah no? What was I thinking?) She said she'd call me back later in the day.

"OH MY GOSH!!!! OPRAH JUST CALLED ME!!!!!!!!!!"

So right when I hung up the phone, Gretchen's call rang back in and she said, "I knew it must have been something important, so I hung on." I informed her Oprah had just called. We laughed. Who would believe it? Gretchen had been with me this whole trek and knew everything. She knew how emotional and sappy I was, and that I actually could just be on

Oprah. (God is downright funny. Oprah called.) After I told her the good news about Oprah phoning, I told her the good news that I was going to live. I shared all of my exhilarating emotions from yesterday with her and we joyously cried together. She then told me "Oh my Gosh! your Neil Diamond song is playing in the background. It's a sign."

I kept having these signs all around me. "What was happening? My voice was getting bigger and bigger and I wasn't even trying. It was just happening! I'm not sure why God chose little ol' me for all this, but I'm thankful for this whole experience." (Now that I know I'm going to live).

I hung up the phone with Gretchen and called Shelley, then Katie, then John. (I knew he wouldn't care so much. He had said to me, "If you're going on Oprah, I'm not going." Party pooper!)

I also logged back on Facebook and friended Megan. I included in her friend request a note telling her to scroll down on my profile page and she would see all of my notes documenting my recent history there. I also changed my Facebook posting to:

> Holly Toner-Rose is "OH MY GOSH!!! OPRAH JUST CALLED!!!!!!!!!!
> Of course, people replied to Oprah.

> Tammy WHA?!!!!!!!!

> Jeremy No way!! Come on holly give all the details~M

> Alisha Holly, remember when you talk to Oprah again, I did help get you on Facebook in the first place. You can have her "friend" me. Thanks!

> John Rose This is getting outta hand.

> Holly Toner-Rose Ok. So I feel I must clarify that it wasn't Oprah herself but it was an employee of Oprah's. That's really

175

the same thing though isn't it? I have Harpo Inc on my caller i.d. Yoohoo!! What a great day!!!

Stacie Shelley called me this afternoon and told me the news....I can't believe it!

Holly Toner-Rose Crazy, crazy day!

Valerie Whoaaa!!! What's the story? We want more details!

Jennifer Details please!

Karyn You have many waiting for details. Holly Michelle please dish!

Holly Toner-Rose Sorry about that ladies. I wrote to Oprah about my experience finding breast cancer through Facebook. Who knows maybe they'll call me back and put me on the show. Wouldn't that be cool?

Holly Toner-Rose Don't forget John you would be sitting right next to me. Hee! Hee!

Having had lunch planned with Carol and Alisha, I drove down to meet them. They were both in their cars on their cell phones, so I tried my best to wait patiently! Carol jumped out of her car first. I was bursting with good news to share. We joked to Alisha that she was spoiling the mood while she was still glued to her phone. She ended her conversation and I did a mini jump (still a little sore) and hollered, "Oprah called me!!!!!!!"

We all jumped up and down, "Oprah called!" Oprah had superseded my wonderful news from my doctor's appointment. We talked for the next fifteen minutes about Oprah calling, what she said, was I going to be on the show, they were going with me etc. I then told them

"Oh I have more good news. I'm going to be okay. I'm going to live! " I relayed to them all the details of my appointment with Dr. Ondreyco and how happy I was. The rest of our lunch we laughed as usual. I felt lucky.

I went home and, of course, I immediately ran and checked Facebook. Megan had accepted my friend request forty-five minutes earlier. I then thought back to the night before, telling Katie how God was giving me this voice. (Again, I really wanted the singing voice.) And here I was now, talking to someone from the Oprah show. I had thought at some point early on that I had a little light in me to shine, and maybe it was someone else's job to shine big. "Who is bigger than Oprah? No one. God works wonders."

Quickly, I went to the laptop and started to find where I had already written about Oprah. I was going to get my book out. It wasn't even my book. This was turning out to be some work of God. Every sign kept moving me this way and that way. I had no control over what was happening. Again, why me? Scrolling through, I concluded she needed to read this whole thing. I know, it probably wasn't the wisest thing to do, but I sent Megan a message. When I went to her Facebook page, up popped a picture of four beautiful little kids. I couldn't help but comment on her babies in my private message through Facebook. "What idiot would act like a psycho by commenting on Megan's babies and say I've got a book? Me!!!!"

While waiting in the car for the girls, I called Shelley. We ran over the conversation minute by minute I had with Megan again. I told Shelley how I couldn't help myself and sent my stupid message. The whole experience kept moving me so I moved with it. Then I called Julie. We laughed. She said, "Oprah will love you." She added, "Oprah will want to be your friend." That was just like Julie. I didn't deserve such huge compliments. I loved her. She always built me up.

The girls got in the car and I screamed, "Oprah called!" They couldn't believe it. We drove home and started the mundane homework routine. The phone rang its double ring, signaling someone out of state was calling.

We all yelled, "OPRAH!" and ran to find a phone. Ivy was the lucky one. She handed me the phone and I felt the need to tell Megan how we ran for the phone.

"Why do I do that?"

She asked me very specific questions about Facebook this time. Was I appreciative for Facebook? How long had I known Shelley? She said they were in the beginning stages of this story and if she had more questions could she call back. I answered this time, "Of course, YES."

Who knows if I'll be on the Oprah show? I somehow think I will. If not, I sure did have fun for the day!

Before I went to bed I called Katie again. She had mentioned if I went on Oprah that I needed to go before I lost my hair. I thought it was interesting. Gretchen had made a comment a few days earlier, when I mentioned I was going to cut my hair short. She said "Oh, Your lovely locks!" Granted, I was aware that I had good hair. I have naturally thick, long, red hair. When I was a kid I hated it. I was called every name in the book. Carrot top, freckle face, Hey Red! (My personal favorite). I was very self-conscious about it and felt inferior for years. There were no redheaded baby dolls, no redheaded Barbies, no redheaded princess' growing up - They were all blonde. I have to admit, even as an adult, I find satisfaction to see Disney's Ariel was a redhead. Silly, I know. Things linger. At some point, I finally decided I liked my hair, maybe I finally decided I liked me. Who knows?

After the "ugly hat" incident, I started grieving for my hair. It's interesting that our whole society would mourn for hair. I had devised several clever plans to hang onto it. First, I was going to have it cut short, turned into extensions and then I could use it later when my hair was growing back. Then I thought I could implant the extensions into hats. I thought that one was brilliant! My last plan was to make my own hair into a wig.

After my appointment with Dr. Ondreyco, I walked and the music filled me with strength once again. I decided to give up my hair that day; I wasn't going to grieve over hair. It was just vanity. It was ego. I wasn't going to hang cling to my ego. It wasn't important. My life was, my kids were, my husband was . . . Not my hair. Even after I had let go of my hair, my friends were now grieving over it.

Lying in bed, I reflected over the day's events. Some friends of John's mom had stopped by that evening with food for us. They were the kindest, happiest couple. After talking for a bit, the wife told us that she had just found out that she had a lump of some kind in her throat. She had a biopsy done that came back unclear, and now she had to have it removed. Her daughter had also just discovered the exact same thing in her body. I realized how selfish I had been. I wasn't the only person going through this. Oh my gosh! They were millions of people at this moment worrying about their lives, their babies, and their husbands. It was the first time this had struck me. I felt rather foolish and completely selfish, for only thinking of me. And here I thought I had to be selfish to get through this. Is that what everyone does during the beginning? I don't think so. Maybe. And my gosh! All of my silly postings on Facebook. Granted, every response lifted my spirits, but what about all of the other people? Maybe those people commenting on me also had people they were close to, suffering from this or worse. My eyes opened a little wider. I choose not to be so ignorant and absorbed in myself.

The next evening our girls wanted to go see Zella Day, the beautiful thirteen-year old girl who sang and played the guitar. She may be the next Hannah Montana. I took the girls and their friends to see her perform outside at the art walk. While watching all of these star struck little girls I saw smiles, headbands, leg warmers, giggles, and sparkling eyes. I saw youth. I saw innocence. I saw dreams forming. While they were mesmerized with Zella I talked to the other mothers there.

After giving a brief update on my status, one mother told me how she was going through something similar. Here she was sending me warm wishes on Facebook, and she was going to be tested for bone cancer soon. She expressed her fears about her babies, her doctors, and her tests. She also told me how she had a choice. Her choice was: to totally stop her life while waiting for her tests months ahead or she could live. She said, "I want to live." I'm with her. You have to live. It struck me again, that there were so many people facing this. I wasn't the only one with fears. I wasn't the only one crying. I wasn't the only one that needed support. I wasn't the only one fighting cancer. It was all around. I drove home listening to the girls giggle. I giggled with them. This was living.

The next day I sat absorbed editing "my book". I ignored my hubby, my kids . . . everything. I spoke with my mother-in-law, Carol, late in the day. She had been in Mexico for the past two weeks. I happily told her my thrilling update. I was more than thrilled that I was going to be okay. I told Carol about her friends, who came to visit me, and how her friend had shared with me her own scares with cancer, and that her daughter was going through the exact same scare with cancer as well. I don't think Carol flinched a bit. I realized then why Carol always said what she said. Her famous motto was, "Onward and Upward." I always thought that she was just a very positive person. Always trying to show the bright side of it all. It was that and so much more. "Onward and Upward." She was just living life. She had seen cancer before, and recovery. She had seen marriage and divorce. She had seen triumph and failure. She had seen birth and death. In life you see it all, but in the end you just keep living. It never stops – for anyone. "Onward and Upward." I was ready to go Onward and Upward.

Yes, I had one more surgery and many treatments to come. I'm sure there will be more ups and downs as well, but isn't that life? Ups and downs. I'm thankful for the ups. My gosh, they are fun! I'm thankful for the downs too. You learn, you appreciate, you grow from each one and the ups just seem that much better.

I lay in bed that night and prayed for all the people struggling. I prayed for God to take away their fears and let them sleep that night. I then realized that my story was over. Not my life, just my story. This was all God wanted me to share - Just a little light. I was ready to live. Live and Give!

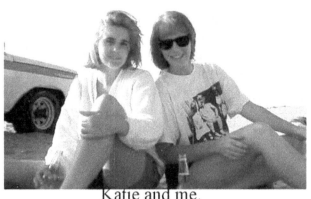

Katie and me.

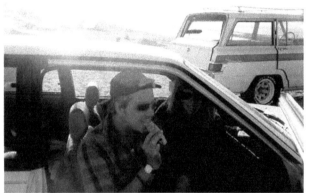

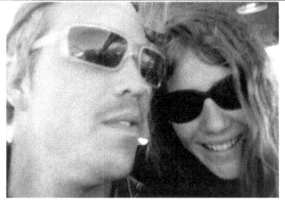

Rocky Point, Mexico 1992
I'm a true believer!

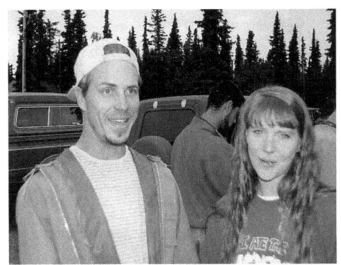

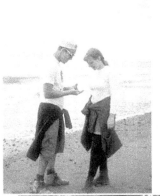

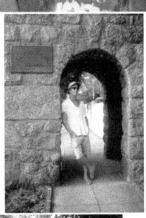

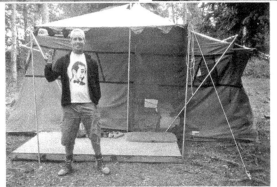

Our summer in Alaska - 1992.

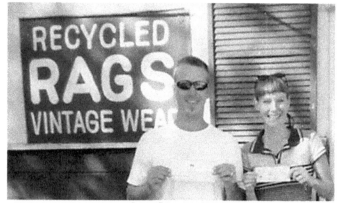
Our first store!

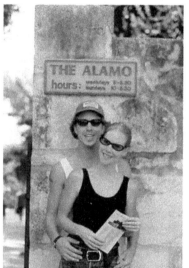

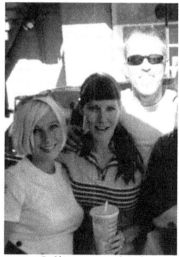
Julie, me and John

Falling
in Love.
The Vegas
Years.
1993-1996

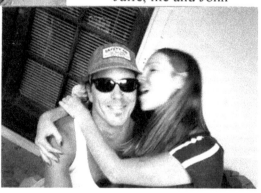

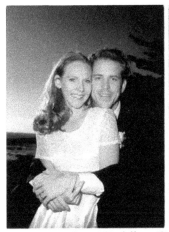
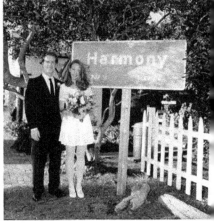

Our Wedding Day - January 21st, 1996.

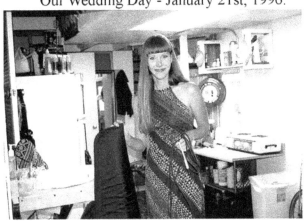

San Diego
The Easy Years
1996-1999.

Above - Me in our 'house'
in the back of our store.
Notice the makeshift
kitchen behind me.

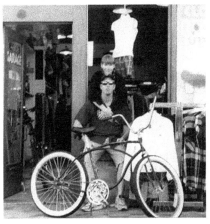

Left - John and me outside
our store 'The Garage'

185

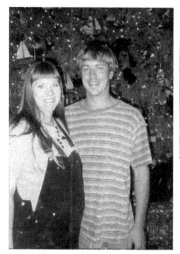
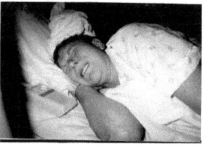

Pregnant, fat and in pain!

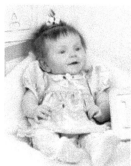
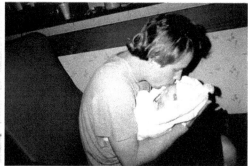

Hannah Michelle Rose 1-03-1998

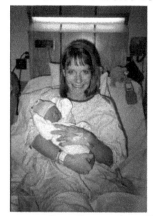
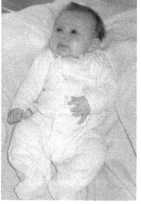

Ivy Lorraine Rose 1-19-1999

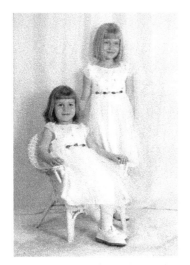
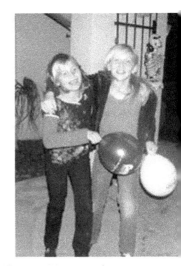
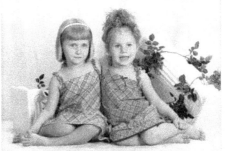

My beautiful babies!

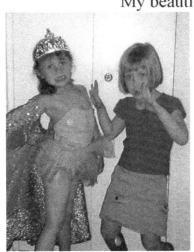
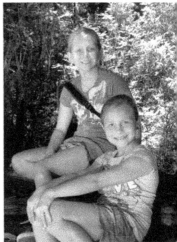

Our Sweet Hannah Banana.

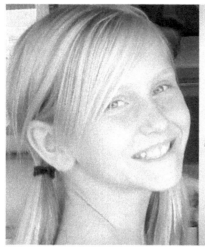
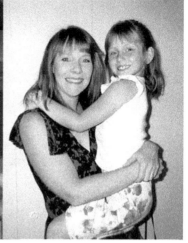
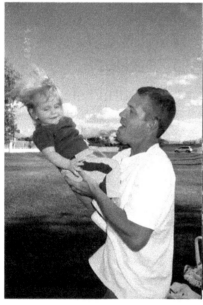
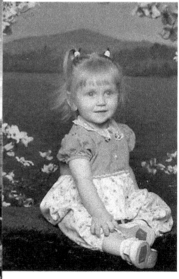

Our Sweet Chavalita Ivy.

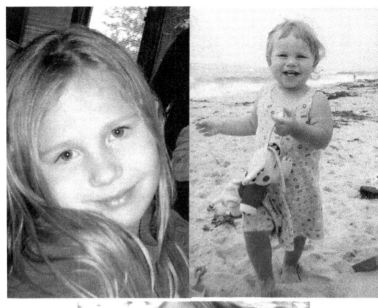

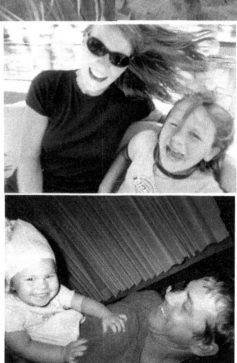

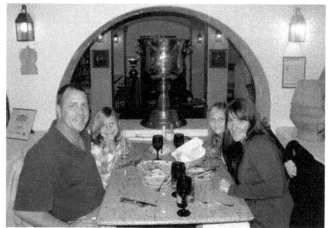

My 39th B-day Dinner.

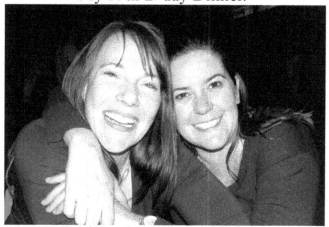

Katie and me on my B-day.

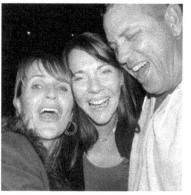

Gretchen, John and me on my B-day.

My last day with hair.

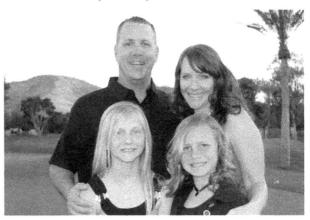

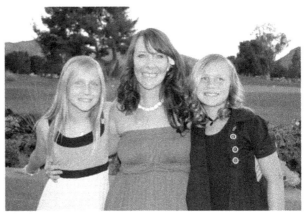

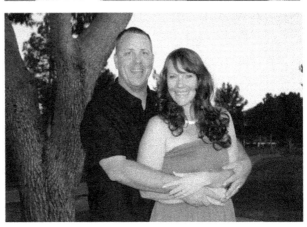

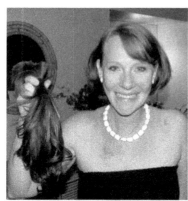

One Step
at a time!

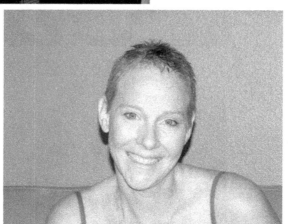

My punk rock buzz.

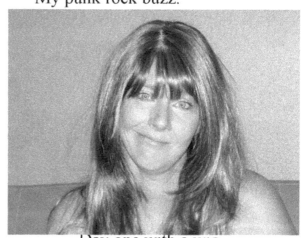

Day one with a wig.

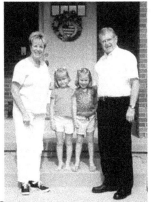
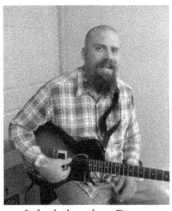

John's mom, Carol & her husband Glenn with the girls.

John's brother Brent.

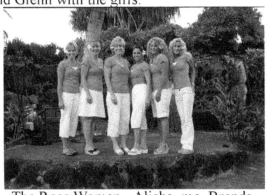

The Rose Women - Alisha, me, Brenda, Margarita, Carol & Teryle.

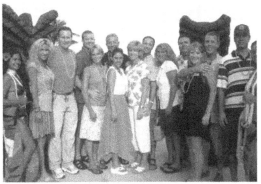

John's family (Teryle, Mark, Stephen, Alisha, Marvin, Margarita, Brenda, Brandon, Carol, Brian, me, John & Danny.

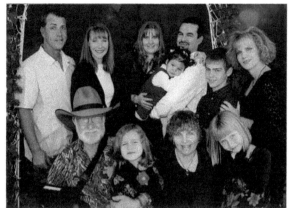

My Family - John, me, Sheree, Gabby, Erik, Shane, Lorie,
John, Ivy, Joan, and Hannah.

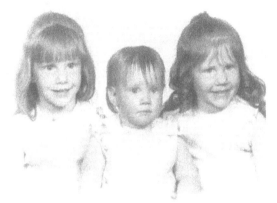

The three little red-heads - Lorie, me, & Sheree.

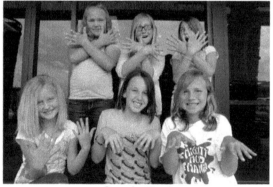

Cousin Fun!

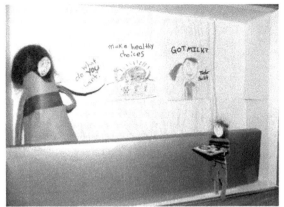

Hannah's fun with human hair.

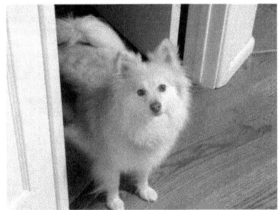

Bobo!

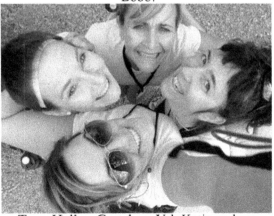

Team Holly - Gretchen, Val, Katie and me.

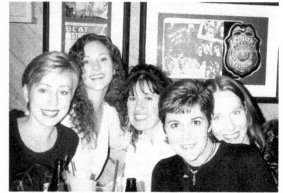

Shelley, Lisa, Krys, Katie and me -199?

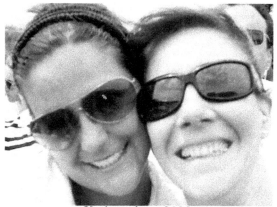

Katie and me 2009

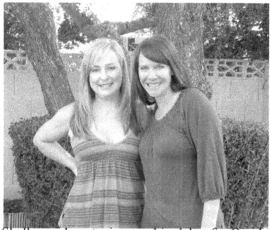

Shelley and me taping our big debut for Oprah.

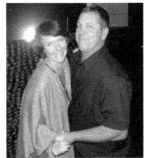
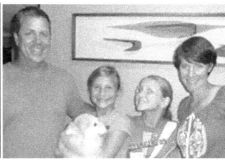

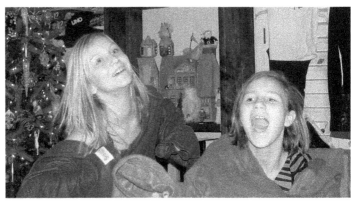

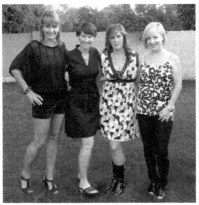

Don't be a Chump!
Check for a Lump! Team.
Gretchen, me, Katie, & Shelley

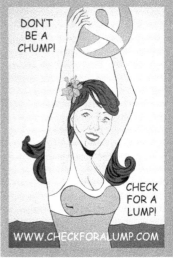

Part II
LIVING AND GIVING
To John and Katie

I struggled with the question whether or not to keep writing. While I was going through the second half of my experience with breast cancer I didn't have the energy physically or emotionally to write anything down, nor did I have any advice to give or any pearls of wisdom to share. My second surgery was awful. No more 'Yays!' No more 'WooHoos!' It was just plain awful. The pain knocked me out. I couldn't do anything afterwards, but sleep. And chemotherapy was downright horrific. I overheard in the chemotherapy room once, that people forget the months they spend during chemo. Having gone through chemotherapy I would rephrase that: they block it out COMPLETELY, because it is too hard on the body, mind and spirit. I'm still not sure I want to relive any of this. Here goes.

Chapter Seventeen

Tuesday, March 9th, 2009. Oprah's staff did indeed call me back. They asked me the details of my story about how Facebook had saved my life. They wanted to know if I would create a short video of myself, and FedEx it to them. "What do you say to Oprah? YES! Never mind that I had surgery scheduled in two days. This was Oprah!"

So, there I was, two days before my second surgery and I added filming for Oprah to my to do list, along with last minute doctor appointments for medical tests.

That afternoon I had a PET scan scheduled. A PET scan -Positron Emission Tomography, would allow a doctor to measure the body's abnormal molecular cell activity to detect any other tumors in my body before treatment. My oncologist needed the results of these tests before I started chemo.

The PET scan procedure was very simple. I sat in a comfy lounge chair while nurses injected radioactive sugar into my veins. After that, I had to sit completely still in a dimly lit room for thirty minutes. During my rest the sugar would attach itself to any cancerous cells in my body. Then the nurse brought me into a large white room where, looming before me was another space age machine, like a miniature rocket, with a huge white sheet of curved metal with a hollow center.

Lying on my back, I was instructed again not to move. I was informed the bed would inch its way through the machine, taking picture after picture of my entire body. The entire process would take approximately twenty minutes. Any possible tumors would light up like a Christmas tree in the pictures.

Throughout the entire procedure my mind was racing with thoughts of Oprah. "I'm going to be on Oprah. How cool is that?" What to wear, what to say, what to do . . . so many

201

exciting details. It was the best distraction I could have asked for that day. My mind wasn't thinking about the chance of tumors and lymph nodes. I was thinking about being on Oprah!

After my test, I frantically ran about trying to accomplish everything before my upcoming surgery. Brenda came over to help clean that afternoon and I invited my brother-in-law Stephen, who was an independent film director, to come over to film me, along with Shelley to help film/edit.

I wanted the filming to be very casual and relaxed. Stephen, being a film director and knowing the filming process wanted professional quality and didn't want me to speak; he advised me to be silent while doing things so they could edit over me. I felt like a complete idiot performing these things in silence. It seemed so unnatural to me and scripted. This wasn't me. So, when he began filming I would speak. I think I drove him crazy all day long. Each clip I couldn't help but to start speaking.

We ended with a shot of me walking down the street. This was something I did in my everyday life, except that today I was dressed up and wearing snappy boots, instead of my usual gym shorts, t-shirt and tennis shoes. I walked down the same street that I had been marching on for months, while listening to Frank Black and convincing myself I was going to beat cancer. I looked into the camera and spoke again. "I used to exercise everyday. Now I walk."

At home we all sat around John's computer and watched our days efforts. When we came to the segment of me strutting down our quiet street in my fancy jeans and boots, we all broke out in laughter. Tears came to our eyes as we held our aching stomachs. We hadn't laughed that hard in years. It was incredibly embarrassing to view and I looked like a complete ass. John and I agreed that if I didn't make it on Oprah the laugh alone was worth it. He was right. That night I posted:

> Holly Toner-Rose has never laughed so hard. I just watched video of myself walking!

<u>Alisha</u> I have never heard John and you laugh so hard. I was laughing at you laughing.

<u>Holly Toner-Rose</u> I thought about it last night lying in bed and started laughing all over again. I woke John up I was laughing so loud.

Thursday, March 12, 2009. Nothing was good that day. John woke up on the wrong side of the bed and was in a bad mood from the moment we left the house. We were on the way to the hospital for my second surgery; more lymph nodes were coming out. I don't know if John was worried about me or worried he had to continue to worry about me. The stress of the past three months was starting to show . . . on both of us.

John and I weren't the only ones having a hard time that day. Arriving at the hospital we sensed that the entire staff was moody. The receptionist couldn't find my chart when I checked in. Her mistake had upset her routine and she transferred her annoyance on to me. Then the admitting clerk was disgruntled as well. She had wrecked her car the evening before and proceeded to tell us all of her complicated frustrations.

There were no smiles, no lucky numbers to make wishes upon, no people from our past administering medicine . . . it was one frown after another. Dr. Zannis was the only one wearing a smile. I guess he was the most important one, since he was the one cutting me open. If I had to choose one person to be smiling that day, it would have been him.

This was my second surgery. I was having an auxiliary lymph node dissection. This procedure is pretty much where a doctor takes a sharp ice cream scooper and excavates all of the lymph nodes from your armpit. Dr. Zannis was performing the second surgery to check if the cancer had spread to any further lymph nodes.

A port was also being placed inside of my right chest. A

port is a triangular piece of plastic the size of a fifty-cent piece, with three small prongs sticking out. The port is placed underneath the skin at your chest and a tube runs from it up to veins in your neck. Drugs/chemo are administered into your body through the port and it allows doctors to gain access to your veins again and again, without causing damage to them.

I awoke from my second surgery. This time I didn't cry out with joy. No "Yay, I'm awake!" This time I cried out in pain. It was excruciating.

"It huuurts. It huuurts." I cried out.

A nurse came over to me "You okay?"

"No, it hurts."

"I've given you all the pain medicine I can give you right now. You'll have to wait a little bit." I asked for John and he came right away.

Soon after Dr. Zannis came by with some general instructions. I had a drip bag connected to me this go around. It was disgusting. The drip bag consisted of a long clear tube, about three feet long, that extended from my left armpit and led to a large clear plastic bulb about the size of a fist and looked kind of like a turkey baster. The bulb's purpose was to collect the bloody fluid that was accumulating in my body. My insides were trying to fill in the many holes that Dr. Zannis had just scooped out of me. John and I were taught to squeeze the bulb every couple of hours to suction out the fluid from my armpit and then empty it. This was gross bloody fluid. This was not going to be fun. He gave us some more details, none of which I can remember. I was in too much pain.

When I arrived home there were no flowers, no cookies, no edible fruit basket . . . Nothing. Apparently, I had used up my sympathy card with the first surgery.

John was still grouchy. I had to ask one by one to have him help me get set up with a blanket, pillow, water, etc. He looked bothered. "Hello, I just had surgery. Was he serious? I couldn't think about why he was sulking at the moment nor did I care because, OH YEAH, I JUST HAD SURGERY!"

That evening, while high on painkillers, I received a call from the staff of the Oprah Winfrey Show with disappointing news. After all our hard work, we didn't make it on Oprah. Late in the evening following surgery a staff member called me and informed me that there was breaking news and they were not going to show our segment. I was still so hazy from all of the painkillers the nurses had injected into me that, when she called, I didn't absorb much of the conversation. The staff member asked me to remove anything I had posted from Facebook regarding Oprah. I passed the information on to John. I didn't check Facebook for a few days, so it wasn't until later that I learned what he posted. I removed his post when I saw it, so I don't have the exact words, but it said something like:

> <u>Holly Toner Rose</u> Who needs Oprah anyway! She's better off without Oprah!

I never would have posted this myself, but I thought it was hilarious. There were a few comments in agreement with John that made me laugh as well.

In my defense and his, "Hello!" I had just had surgery. I was doped up on painkillers and Oprah's staff gave me instructions to follow that entailed getting off of the couch. I wasn't able to move from my couch, or even able to, had I wanted, let alone coherent enough to follow instructions. And had they known my hubby, they would have realized he would most definitely post something rebellious and comical about the situation. I didn't think about it or care. I took my pain pills and slept.

The following day after surgery I slept for the entire day. Occasionally, I would wake up in pain and take more medicine. I was not prepared for the pain. My entire left side was completely bandaged up. I didn't care to see what was underneath the bandages just yet. Maneuvering my body enough to reach them was out of the question anyway. I was not able to move my left arm – at all. This also made resting extremely difficult. There was no way in hell I could lay on my left side (the side Dr. Zannis had cut open). Lying on the right side was impossible too! Lying on my stomach was absolutely absurd. My only other option was lying on my back. This was only made tolerable by placing an oversized pillow underneath my arm for support, along with taking some powerful pain pills.

The intense suffering came as a shock. This was nothing like my first surgery. There was no relief from the pain either. Even after taking pain pills it still hurt, so I took more to sleep and escape the pain.

When I woke, I would call out to John. He had to help me to the bathroom. Every step I took was agonizing and left me weak. I couldn't move my arm further than an inch from my side. John had to pull my pants up and down, and then stand next to me holding my drip bag in his hand. He also had to detach the drip bag and empty the bloody contents into the toilet and reattach it. I had never been so helpless in my life. Never.

Three days later I was still in excruciating pain and was beginning to stink. I had been wearing the same clothes for three days. Just the thought of having to change clothes was stressful. My spirits were falling and I needed something to pick me up. I thought a shower might do the trick. Fresh body, fresh clothes, fresh mind . . . It didn't work.

Tears of pain streamed down my face while John undressed me. Incapable of moving my arm John bathed me. He washed my hair with loving hands and tenderly scrubbed my body as I stood helplessly crying. He looked at me lovingly and soothed, "Oh Momo! It's going to be okay."

I cried out, "It huurts. It huurts."

"I'll take care of you honey." And he did. He bathed me, dressed me and loved me. Back to the couch I went.

Ready to type my troubles away, I tried setting up my

laptop, but no luck. My arm was not willing to participate. It was just too painful. "This isn't fair. It's not fair! Why do I have to go through this? Why God? Why me?" I sobbed.

Chapter Eighteen

Hannah and Ivy had their spring break coming up that week - One whole week off of school. They deserved some fun and entertainment after the past couple of months of stress (we all did). There was no way I could do anything to entertain them in this state. Usually, I made sure they had fun activities planned for any breaks and I loved being a part of it.

I remembered past vacations taking the girls to visit KK in California. Visiting Katie was always a treat. She was the best hostess, with special treats for all of us and dolls to play with and musical instruments to strum and adventurous stories to hear.

While visiting Katie we usually made our way down to the beach. Ivy loved the beach. As a baby we had to watch her very carefully because she was ready to dive right into the ocean. She had no fear. She still doesn't.

Hannah, on the other hand, had a love/hate relationship with the beach. When we lived in San Diego she would beg me everyday to take her to the beach. I would oblige her and stroll her and Ivy blocks down the steep path to the beach. Immediately, upon stepping foot into the sand Hannah would cry out that she wanted to return home. Once the sand gathered on her little hands and feet, you could see the frustration building up on her face. Frantically, she fought to keep the sand off of her, but it was a losing battle. We usually left the beach soon after arriving, to go home and clean away the tiny particles of sand from her little body.

I also had a love/hate relationship with the beach. I loved the ocean, the waves, the sun, the fun . . . I hated that I had to expose myself in a bathing suit in public. I still hadn't gotten over my body dysmorphia. I think it was part of my obsessive nature. Funny thing is, though, I think the beach or maybe it was my babies who helped me get over it.

I distinctly recall one year going to the beach, just the girls and me. As I sat on my beach towel fretting over the fact that people were going to see my big fat imperfect body, I suddenly realized what was really important. I realized that my babies were not going to have fun sitting on the towel all day with me. They wanted to play in the ocean – with me! At this point they were too young to get close to the ocean without me. What did I want them to remember? Mommy sitting on some towel worried and fretting that people would notice her imperfections or Mommy jumping in the waves with them? I wanted them to remember having fun with me. I bravely took off my clothes to bare my bathing suit, saddle bags and all. I held my babies' hands and we jumped and laughed as the waves came tumbling down on us. There were going to be no waves this year. This year I would be sitting on the couch.

Alisha called and invited the girls to go to Utah to visit John's mother for the week. Alisha was always thinking of others. She kept telling me that I was inspiration to her, but really she was an inspiration. She was so helpful and kind.

Hannah already had a trip planned for the first couple of days so we decided to let Ivy go to Utah. It was Ivy's first big trip away from home.

During that quiet week I lay on the couch and I found excitement and escape thinking about my book. Something was supposed to happen with my book. It was just as Katie had said, "The world was conspiring with me to make it happen," – it was supposed to happen.

> Holly Toner-Rose finished her book today
> about her journey the past two months. I
> can't wait for everyone to read it. You're
> all in there. Anyone know a publisher?

I needed another opinion on my book. Who to ask though? It was scary to put yourself out there for rejection. That was something I didn't normally do. Residing within me

209

was a deep fear of rejection.

I was confident that my book was good though. Ready to take the big test I asked Janeen to read it. She was so blunt and honest. I could count on her to give me an honest opinion. Everyone else that read it might feel obligated to tell me they liked it only because I had cancer. Not Janeen. She would tell me the truth - the honest truth.

When she came by to check in on me that morning, I asked her if she would do me the honor. As I handed her my printed copy my head screamed, "Don't do it. Don't put yourself out there." I stamped out the voice inside me and let go.

For the entire day I wondered what Janeen thought about my book. "Was she not calling me because she thought it was awful and didn't know how to tell me? What? I thought it was good. Crap! What made me think I could write a book? I'm going to look like an idiot. Wait! It is good. I know it is good. It wasn't just me that poured on to those pages, somehow it was God as well. How could it not be good with His input?"

That evening, while checking my Facebook I found a message from Janeen. I opened the message to find:

> Janeen I am not done with the book yet... but I just had to say I love it so much. I have been laughing and crying all along. Then I just got to the 11:11 2:22 3:33 part and I almost fell off my chair. The last few times I was with Danny He told me every time he looks at the clock he says it is always the same 3 or 4 numbers mom and it freaks me out! I never knew about the wish. I cannot wait to tell him.... But I thought OH MY GOD maybe he is supposed to make a movie about you and your experience. maybe for his school thesis. With facebook and all as part of it I think it really appeals to a large audience

210

and health care and breast cancer awareness and all that ..I am going to tell him about it. Maybe he can read it when you are ready and maybe he will make a movie.....It would be such a good message...Who knows we may all be at the Oscars all because of you and your boobies. . .love you...I feel like I have been in your head all day and night. I will call tomorrow after I am done with your wonderful book!!!!

"She liked it!!! Yay! She liked it!!!!!"

Monday, March 16, 2009. Today I had my Muga test, Multiple Gated Acquisition scan. This would take a look at my heart in motion at every angle, to make sure my heart was strong enough to withstand chemo. I was still in pain so John drove me to my appointment.

The Muga test was fascinating. First, the technician injected a substance into me that was not from the planet earth. Seriously! It was from another planet!!!! In my body!!!!! Crazy!!!

After my injection I was placed onto another flat bed with a machine that looked out of this world as well. It had a large wall of metal that rotated around me taking pictures.

The technician told me fascinating stories about his hometown while the robotic machine moved inch-by-inch taking pictures. He was from Athens, Ohio and he recalled wondrous nights out seeing all of the great 80's bands performing in small clubs.

Our conversation brought me back to my college days at NAU. They were some of the best years of my life. So many moments from NAU will be forever branded in to my memory:

dancing all night to the b-52's in Tinsley hall, singing backup to Val belting out Aretha Franklin tunes, watching the sunrise over the dome, "The Dome!", Alpine Pizza – too many memories there to just mention one, Grasshopper point, Sunshine Bakery, The Mad I, the Barracks, Snowbowl, the Monte Vista . . . Life was full of fun then. It was also full of friends I treasured. I cherish my college days at NAU and all of the wonderful people who were a part of it.

Time flew by as I sat reminiscing and before I knew it my test was completed. On my way out the door the technician told me, "Oh by the way, you are radioactive for another six hours. Be sure to stay at least an arm's length from your children. Nothing has been proven, but to be on the safe side stay away from your daughters."

Arriving at home I warned Hannah to keep back. With every step around the house, I held my arms out in front of me, to protect her from harm.

> <u>Holly Toner-Rose</u> is radioactive for another 6 hours. Stay back!

The next few days I spent alone on the couch. John helped entertain Hannah and her friends. He took them to the St. Patrick's Day parade. I watched them all leave excitedly. I watched my life passing me by.

"This isn't fair. I want to go. I want to be with them. I want to have fun. This sucks. Cancer Sucks!!!" I took another pain pill and slept the day away.

The following day I decided I wasn't going to wallow any longer. I was going to keep living. Needing to get off of the couch and out of the house, I opted to try to go for a walk. Walks had been helpful the past two months. The sunshine touched me with its happy rays and the fresh breeze blew off some of my sorrows.

I left the house in high spirits. One house – "My arm hurts." Two houses, "Crap this hurts." Three houses, " I can do this." Four houses, "Oh my gosh! This hurts!!!" Five houses,

"Who am I kidding?" I slowly inched my way back home. Back to the couch. Tomorrow, I thought, "I'll go ten houses." When I returned home I posted:

> Holly Toner-Rose is I think I'll go for a walk for outside now, the sunshine is calling my name.

People were always there on Facebook to cheer me on.

> Valerie "just can't stay inside all day, gotta get out get you some of those rays...!"

> Holly Toner-Rose I was wondering who would catch that.
> I'm doing good. I just made it out 5 houses and back. Hip hip hooray!

> Matt Have a very Brady day, cuz!

> Jeanne "everybody's smilin', Sunshine Day!!" It's a happy day! I'm glad you got out!

> Vicki yay!!!

March 18th, 2009. It was the day after St. Patrick's Day. John and I met on this day seventeen years ago. It was my college spring break of 1992. I had transferred from NAU to ASU in Tempe, Az. I had just been fired from my waitressing job across town because I no longer had transportation to get to and from work. I had been in a car wreck that totaled my car and had to wait a few weeks for it to be fixed. Really, though, they fired me because I was always late, and not the best waitress to begin with.

I applied all around my college campus for a new waitress job. I was waiting to hear back from someone-anyone when Katie called me. She was up from Tucson and wanted me to go to Rocky Point, Mexico with her for the weekend. With hesitation in my voice I told her, "Katie, I can't go. I don't have a job. I don't have any money. I can't."

She convinced me in her gruff Katie tone, "It's not like you have a job to go to or anything. You might as well go have some fun while you can. When you get back you're going to have to start working again and then you won't be able to take off of work. Besides, I won't be here to go with since I'm leaving for New York soon." And so I packed my bag and off to the beach we went.

Gin Blossoms was blaring out of the stereo throughout the four-hour drive. We arrived in Rocky Point to a sea of scattered cars on the beach. This was back in the day when there were no hotels on the beach, no showers, no condos, no luxuries . . . You slept in your car, on the sand near a campfire, or if you were really lucky you pitched a tent. That was a weekend in Rocky Point back then. It consisted of the beach, the bar and boys.

When we arrived we made no hesitation and headed over to The Reef bar ready to begin our vacation. With icy cold Coronas in hand, we decided to venture down the beach and take a look around. Katie and I both donned our cut off Levi's that we frayed ourselves with band t-shirts tucked in. We chatted as we made our way down the sand path when I noticed two boys coming head on. One was as cute as could be. He had a swagger to his step. He was wearing a green striped vintage sixties tank with jean shorts-most likely his Girbaud shorts from back in the day. His hair was blond and wavy and somewhat layered giving him a sexy, "I don't give a damn" rebellious look that I loved so much. He was hot!!!

Katie and I smiled as they passed us by and he nonchalantly uttered out, "A red-head." My heart fluttered, but we were way too cool (really too shy and insecure - at least I was) to stop and we kept going. We made our way to the beach patio and took a seat.

I saw a few friends I knew, so we started chatting with them. A little time went by and low and behold here came blondie boy strutting up the path. He was striking and manly and My Oh My!

He knew the guys we were talking with, in fact, he was camping right next to them. We all joked and laughed and drank our Coronas. Hours later the sun was starting to set and it was time to regroup for the night. As Katie and I started to head out they asked us if we wanted to join their camp. This was not unusual for Rocky point. It was typical to pull your car up on the beach next to your friends. And so we did.

Katie and I went to the car to repark. We quickly pulled out the make-up, touched up, brushed, and did the traditional flip of the hair to fluff it up. After fixing ourselves up as best we could in the confines of our car we drove over to their camp and parked for the night. I was anxious and eager to hang out with John with some more. He was fascinating!

We hopped out of the car and went over to the booming campfire. John was nowhere in sight. "Where did he go? Where did he go?" The night went on and my mind still kept coming back to John. "Where did he go?" I looked for him at every turn and every man passing by I hoped it was him returning.

As the evening went on, one of John's friends kept hitting on me. I was not interested in his friend. I was interested in John. I decided to go for a walk hoping to avoid having to hurt the guy's feelings. I thought he might just forget about me if I left for a while, that or pass out.

While making my escape I found John. He had been fast asleep in his truck. He was just now waking up. I was so excited to find him. I had been thinking about him non-stop from the moment I saw his blonde hair blowing in the ocean breeze.

John and I were talking away when his friend came looking for me. Nervously my mind raced, "I'm not interested in this other guy. I wish he would just leave me alone. I don't want him to start flirting with me and definitely not in front of John. John may lose interest if he thinks his friend is interested in me. I like John. This other guy needs to leave. LEAVE ME ALONE!"

215

Panicked, not knowing what else to do to escape John's friend, I climbed into John's truck. I looked at John nervously, sure he must be thinking, "What the hell is this girl doing?" He smiled. And I smiled back. We continued our conversation, ignoring his friend completely. Finally his friend got the hint and disappeared. I don't think we even noticed his absence, since we were too enthralled with each other. From that point on we became inseparable. It was fate. It was true love.

Now here I was seventeen years later still in love with my hubby. He was still by my side. We had been through a grueling three months. We were both tired and scared, but I was the only one who had been allowed to show it. I had many breakdowns during the course of my cancer treatment. John only had one. Please keep that in mind as you read the next part of my story.

Friday, March 20, 2009. I was still incapable of taking care of myself. I couldn't bathe myself, cook for myself or really tend to myself at all. I was utterly and completely helpless. Not only was I feeling physically down, I was also emotionally down. My idea of a quick recovery had flown out the window, in a gust, days ago. My girls were away, having fun and living life without me. Life was passing me by as I sat on the couch recovering and there wasn't a damn thing I could do about it. I was helpless.

I'm guessing John was drained at this point as well. He had been taking care of me, the girls, himself, and the house. His brother Danny called and invited him to the Rockabilly festival that weekend. I was excited for John to go out and have some fun. He could go let loose and not think about me or cancer for a few hours. He needed that. He deserved to have some fun. His plan was just a bit different from my plan.

My thoughts were that John was leaving that evening. Obviously, I couldn't take care of myself for the whole day.

Hannah was gone. Ivy was gone. I was relying on John to take care of me. I hadn't showered in days and I was starting to smell again. The pain of moving my arm to take off my clothes was excruciating, so during my healing time I only showered when it was absolutely necessary. I asked John if he could help me shower before he left.

It was late that Friday morning, when a man appeared at our house to fix our cable. Still incapacitated and sitting on the couch I watched the cable man go about his business fixing this and that when I heard John's phone ring. A couple minutes later he informed me he was leaving soon. I assumed he had talked to his work. (I had assumed wrong).

John paced about, antsy to leave the house. "I gotta get going Holly," he said very bluntly. My eyes widened and I looked at the cable man then back at John then back to the cable man and my eyes grew even bigger.

I was not able to move more than an inch without being in pain and John wanted to leave me alone with the cableman in our house. John huffed at my terrified glance. "Was he kidding me? I just had surgery. It's not like he's never late to work! Like he can't wait fifteen @#$*&!# minutes for this guy to finish."

"I've got to leave Holly. I'm gonna be late."

He obviously didn't read my panicked look of, "Please don't leave me here alone with this man in our house while I am helpless!" so I asked him point blank "Can you wait?" with both fear and bitterness in my voice. He dramatically huffed and puffed some more. I didn't think I was asking too much. I was only asking him to wait a little bit longer while keeping with his wife company WHO JUST HAD SURGERY!!!!!!

The cable man finally finished the job and left. John argued that I was being impossible. Angrily he asked, "Why couldn't you have just sat with the cable man? What is the big deal?"

"I CAN'T MOVE, JOHN. I don't want to be here

HELPLESS, with a MAN I don't KNOW who is MISSING a TOOTH. I don't think I'm asking too much here."

He wound up storming out of the house and I sat there on the couch crying. Crying because I was mad. Crying because I was in pain. Crying because I didn't want any of this anymore! And then the phone rang. It was John's brother Danny. Danny was wondering if John had left to meet him at the rockabilly festival.

Fuming, I thought to myself, "He wasn't even going to work. He was rushing out on me to go the festival. All I wanted was for him to wait with me. Maybe help me take a shower before he left. I didn't even care that he was going out for the night. I wanted him to go have fun. I just didn't think he was going to leave me ALL DAY LONG!!!!!!!"

Trying to distract myself from my anger I watched more comedy series, another present from Alisha. It worked for a while. What I really needed was a shower though. John could have at least offered to help me shower before he left. He knew I couldn't do that alone right now.

Cheering myself on, "I can do this. I don't need him to take care of me. Damn it! I can take care of myself. I'm not going to sit here and feel sorry for myself. I can do this. I can!"

Slowly, I inched my way off of the couch and wobbled into the bedroom. Standing in the closet out of the mirror's harm, I began lifting up my shirt. "Oh my gosh! This hurts! This hurts! I can't do this!" Fighting with myself to keep going I persisted "You can do this Holly! Just like a band-aid. One swoop and it will be over. You can do this!" With strength from above, my arm lifted, pulling at every stitch that Dr. Zannis had carefully sewn. "OOOOWWWW!" I cried out sobbing. "OOOOWWWW!" I had never felt anything so painful in my life. And I did it!

Walking past the mirror my curiosity got the best of me and I stole a glance at my underarm. "OH MY GOSH! I CAN'T LOOK AT THAT. IT'S HUGE!!!! OH MY

GOSH!!!!!!!" As quickly as I could, I hobbled into the shower ready to wash away my tears.

The wound I saw was no small scar. It was four inches long and it looked like a baboon's butt, pink and puffy, stretching across my armpit. Sobbing more I cried out, "This hurts. It hurts. Why God? Why me? This isn't fair. And why did John leave me? He left me! I'm totally helpless here and he left me!"

The shower wasn't so successful. Moving my arm was out of the question, so soap didn't make it any where near my left side. The pain was just too intense. It wasn't worth it. And since I couldn't move my left hand, washing my right side was tricky in itself. I did what I could. Mostly, I cried.

Turning off the water, I thought I would be turning off the sorrow too, only to find out it had just began. I hadn't given any thought to after the shower. Cold and shivering I cried out, "What was I thinking? Damn it! I can't even dry myself off!" Picking up a towel with my right hand I dabbed away at the water still running down my body. "Why was I so stupid???? I can't do this by myself!!!!! Sure Holly. You don't need anybody. You can do this. DAMN IT!!! I CAN'T!!!!! How the hell am I going to get dressed?" Standing in front of my dresser naked with a shirt in my hand I sobbed. And I sobbed. I was utterly helpless. I had never in my thirty-nine years of life felt so completely helpless and alone. It was a terrifying.

After what seemed like an eternity I thought to myself there must be a way around this. I can dress myself somehow. Looking in my closet I scanned shirt-by-shirt visualizing how I could put each one on, when I came to a camisole that I wore underneath sheer shirts. It was kind of like a tube top. I could put it on like a tube top from the bottom up. I shimmied my way into the top. It took a few minutes and a few more tears but I did it. "Damn it."

Heading back to the couch, utterly exhausted, I was ready for a nap. After a few hours of sleep I decided to call John. I wanted him back home with me. I needed him by my side. I needed him.

Carol, Brian's wife, called me at that point. I recounted my sad story to Carol, recalling every pathetic detail and how I was angry with John. She reminded me that John had been there every minute for me, the past couple of months. He stood proud and tall all of these months never once complaining. She convinced me he deserved a little bit of a break.

Not quite ready to reprieve him I put myself to sleep in Ivy's room. I wanted nothing to do with John that evening. I was deeply hurt by his actions. I lay in bed and prayed to God. I prayed that I could forgive him for leaving me alone that day and not taking care of me.

I don't think God had heard my prayers just yet when John came home. When John arrived we fought about the events of the day. I ran back to Ivy's room and once more pulled the covers over my bruised body and spirit, and I prayed. I prayed that I would forgive John. This time God did hear me. I thought about how strong John had been the previous two months. How he walked around our house knowing I had cancer for an hour without telling me. How he never showed me his fears or tears. I thought about how wonderful he was. What a great man he really was and what a great father he was to our girls. Carol was right. He just had a moment of weakness. I had my moments too. I had no right to judge him! He didn't deserve that. Plus, I loved him.

Chapter Nineteen

March 23rd, 2009. I was scheduled for my meeting with chemo-nurse. The nurse was going to walk us through the steps of my chemotherapy treatment ahead of me; tell me what to expect, where to go and what to do. While driving out of our neighborhood to my appointment I glanced at the mountain ahead of me. Dreamily I thought, "Two months ago I was steadily hiking up that trail. I was strong and confident. Now I am headed for chemo. One day I will climb that mountain again." I reached out for John's hand and he was there.

Twenty minutes later we were seated in my oncologist's office. My nurse, Mary, called my name. She was a tall, soft-spoken woman. She escorted us into small room with a desk and two chairs. We sat down, and frightened, I reached for John again. I didn't want to hear any of this. I didn't want to be here. I didn't want to have chemo.

She went over the basics with us. I asked her if everyone loses their hair. She said that with the type of chemo I was doing, I was guaranteed to lose all of my hair, and all of body hair as well. Upon hearing this my spirits sank even more.

Next, Mary opened up a laptop with a movie for us to watch. The movie was basically one of those commercials you see on TV, selling you on the benefits of the medicine and then protecting themselves by listing every last possible side effect one could encounter.

The benefits were obvious. Chemo was going to kill every last cancer cell in my body. It was going to allow me to live cancer free. The list of side effects was never-ending. It started out with slight nausea, headache, and body aches. And it kept going with tingling of the hands and feet, blisters inside your mouth, and weight loss and possible anorexia.

John and I started to giggle after a minute as it continued on with possible heart attack, loss of hair, and bone pain and we laughed some more. The list became more and more ridiculous with gangrene, loss of limbs and death. It was absolutely comical. We laughed harder and harder with each passing minute and then we were laughing that we laughing. I can only imagine what the staff outside our room must have thought. I'm guessing they usually heard cries coming from that room instead of echoing bolts of hysterical laughter.

At one point during the long segment of side effects, reality crept in, overwhelming me with fears. "Loss of limbs. Are they serious?" I looked at John, fearful, and he mirrored my look. My eyes cried, "This is chemo - Crap! This is really happening." Lovingly, he smiled at me, taking away my fears, and we laughed some more.

After our video, we were given the grand tour of the chemo room. As we entered, fear came running back to me. I looked about. Everyone was old - Everyone! "Why am I here? Crap, I have to have chemo. This isn't happening." I greedily grabbed John's arm. "I'm not supposed to be here. I'm not supposed to have cancer!"

Mary, my nurse, informed me that she would make sure to schedule herself in the chemo room for my first visit, so I could see a familiar face. I didn't want to hear or see anymore of the chemo room. I just wanted out of there. I wanted out quickly. I wasn't ready for chemo. Not today.

I called Katie and told her about our appointment. I told her "Good news is I might get anorexia for a few months. I'm shooting for that side effect instead of gangrene. Wouldn't that be nice? It could be the best diet ever, without even trying." We laughed as usual.

I was so thankful that Katie had moved back from Barbados a year ago. We decided it had been fate, her moving back. Little did we know that I would get breast cancer soon after she moved back. Besides John, Katie was my main support. She took on the job of cheering me up. She called me every day. Her fulltime job for months was making me laugh. I would call in the morning and say, "Okay, I need a funny story." And sure enough she would pull something out for me to laugh at. She was and is an amazing friend. I am lucky to have a friend like her for the past twenty-five years.

Ivy returned home from Utah that evening. I had missed her so much. She excitedly told us about her trip with Aunt Alisha and her cousins. I was so happy for her that she enjoyed herself. Ivy deserved some fun. She had been scared for too long. At the same time I felt a tinge of remorse and envy; envy of Alisha who was there to share it with her and remorse for having to miss it. Ivy was home. It was comforting to have our family all together again. I loved them all so much.

Wednesday, March 25th, 2009 - It was the day before my first chemo appointment. I tired to keep my spirits high. I picked myself up and walked on. I listened to Frank Black as I marched on, "I can do this. I can do this." My arm still hurt but I was going to walk on. "You can keep your ego, Cancer. I'm still here and I'm going to beat you." I looked over at the mountain and thought to myself, "Damn it! I want to be walking up that mountain again. I don't want to do this anymore! Why me? I'm scared. Damn it! I'm scared." I tried to hold back the tears with little luck.

I was strolling down Moon Valley lane with tears rolling down my cheeks. As I turned the corner I noticed Janeen and Leslie happily chatting away. I wasn't up for this. Not today. I didn't want to put on a happy face right now. I couldn't. As I approached they both smiled at me and asked how I was. My mask instantly appeared and I cheered how well I was doing. Then it came. The question.

Leslie asked, "When do you start chemo?"

My lip quivered as I let out, "Tomorrow." Then I poured out my fears to Janeen and Leslie. I couldn't have held it in if I had wanted to. "I'm scared. I'm scared," I cried. They put their arms around me and they cried too. With tears still streaming down I said hopeful, "Maybe it won't be so bad. Maybe it's just the word that is scary. Right?"

Janeen chimed in her most upbeat voice "It probably won't be that bad. You're going to get through this. That is all there is to it. YOU are going to get through this." I was still scared.

After my walk I proceeded to get ready for my big appointment with Dr. Zannis. We were going to find out the results of my last surgery today. The lymph nodes that he had removed had been sent to the lab for testing to determine if the cancer had spread. Today we would find out my fate.

I held John's hand tightly as we drove there. "Crap! What if it spread? I had been so consumed with the pain that I wasn't thinking I still had cancer in me." John was convinced that Dr. Zannis had taken it all out of me and it was gone. That was that. I hadn't thought about it until now.

We were ushered back to a room soon after check in. I nervously looked at John. His smiling eyes gave me confidence that I was going to be okay. Dr. Zannis came in with a smile on his face. Holding my chart in his hand he cheered, "Good news! All fourteen lymph nodes came back clean." He then explained that he had to tell some women sitting in front of him that all of their lymph nodes had come back cancerous. He told us how lucky we were. We were lucky. I knew that (I remind myself everyday how lucky I am). Dr. Zannis wished us well and gave us a congratulatory hug. I was going to be okay.

This wasn't going to be so bad. I now just had to survive chemo and radiation, and then all of this would be over.

The reality that I was going to loose my hair still filled

me with dread. Everyone repeatedly recommended that I purchase my wigs before I lost my hair. They said it wouldn't be so devastating if I had the wigs in advance (they were wrong).

I needed someone there with me to get me through it. This was a girlfriend's job - not John's. Gretchen was so upbeat and positive I knew she would be comforting to me. She could keep my spirits up. She met me later that day for wig shopping.

We walked into Wig Heaven. There were blonde wigs, black wigs, red wigs, short wigs, longs wigs, afro wigs, partial wigs, scarves, hats and more. I picked up several wigs and put them back down. Looking at Gretchen with a hint of sorrow in my eyes she perked right up and said, "Here's a sassy one Holly! I got to tell you I'm kinda jealous. You're going to have so much fun with wigs. Look at these. You're going to be hot!" I knew Gretchen was the right one to bring with me.

I sat at the hair station with Gretchen on one side and the owner of the store on the other side. I tried on wig after wig. The first one was okay. The second was awful. The third actually looked a little like me, just the wrong color. We scanned swatches of hair color trying to match it to my natural hair. Finally we found a match. The wig looked like me. It even had a part in the hair. Wigs with parts were approximately $200 more. I was willing to pay for the part. I wanted to look like me, not me with a wig.

As the owner wrote down the order for my first wig, I tried on more. Gretchen brought me piles of stuff to try on. I tried on a short dark bob, it had deep shades of red and almost a purplish hue to it. It was fun. My mind perked up thinking, "Okay, I can have fun with this. This won't be so bad. Fun with wigs!"

Next she dressed my head with a scarf and said, "This might be kind of cute. I like that." I looked at the scarf on my head that covered every last strand of hair I had.

Sad thoughts rushed out, "I'm going to be bald. I don't want to be bald. I look ugly. I'm going to be bald and ugly. Why? It's not fair. Why? I DON'T WANT TO BE BALD." Gretchen looked into my eyes and saw my sadness. Quickly, she grabbed the scarf off of my head and picked up the sassy wig I liked.

"Back to hair. Back to happy!" she exclaimed as she clapped her hands. And she did bring me back to happy.

In the end I wound up with the long red wig, a short sassy bob, and a long blonde one. As I checked out, Gretchen grabbed one of the scarves that I tried on. She wanted to buy it for me to keep my little head warm at night just in case. She was so thoughtful and kind.

I made it. I had my wigs. Now I just had to wait for the hair to fall out. (Wah!!!!!!)

Holly Toner-Rose had a ball shopping for wigs. I will be lookin' sassy!

I prayed that night, "Please God give me the strength to get through this. Please." John held me tight and I cried myself to sleep in his arms.

Chapter Twenty

Thursday March 26th, 2009. Today was chemo number one. I woke up feeling a little nervous. "I can do this. I can do this." I cheered myself on. John drove me to the oncologist. Nervously, I stroked his hand for comfort the entire drive. Somehow, me touching him always calmed me, his hand, his arm, his chest . . . Didn't matter which part, just connecting to his skin healed me. It had been that way since the day we met. He was so strong and manly and he took care of me. He somehow took away all of my fears and insecurities just by being near him. No one else had ever done that. He made me feel special in every way.

Heading in I toted everything I thought I would possibly need. I brought books, Sudoku puzzles and pens, thank you cards to fill out, John's laptop so I could work on my book, Jolly Ranchers (someone told me they help take away the bad taste of chemo), and, the most important thing - John. They allowed one person to sit with you in the chemo room on the your first round of chemo. After that you were on your own. John had planned to stay with me the whole day while I sat through chemo.

I checked in and sat down. As I looked across the room I still couldn't believe this was happening to me. I recalled how I had sat in this very office years ago for a check-up on my Leiden Factor V blood condition. At that time, I remember looking at the elderly patients, feeling sorry for them because they were so sick. I didn't look like I belonged in that office, not then and not now. But here I was starting chemo. I just hoped I would be alive at their age.

A few minutes passed and we were called back. The room was a Southwest pink hue with bright hospital lightning. On my left there was a long row of Lazy-Boy style chairs backed up against the wall lined up on my left. Another longer line on my right backed up against a wall of windows allowing in a glimmer of sunlight. Each Lazy Boy was dressed in blue vinyl with a reclining lever on one side.

The nurse who ushered me back advised me to, "pick a chair, any chair." My eyes darted back and forth along each row. I didn't want to make anyone feel uncomfortable looking at them so I tried to be quick. "God, everyone looks so sick. Am I going to look that way after today? Crap, I don't want to do this. Why?"

Nurses went past me this way and that. I choose a chair at the end of the row. I had a window view - woohoo. John sat down next to me on a stool and we held hands.

The nurse Mary came in and calmly said, "Hello." She had scheduled herself in the chemo room that day, just as she had promised. She brought me a large fluffy white pillow and a white cotton sheet to drape over myself. The sheet was warm and toasty like it had just been pulled out of the dryer. She rolled in the IV holder and placed two large clear baggies full of clear liquid on it. Each bag had a long clear tube connected to it that would soon be connected to me.

The first step was to take some of my blood to test the levels to ensure my counts were good. If all was well, they would then proceed with the next step of hooking up my port. In order to do this the nurse, would first apply a cold spray to my chest where my port was placed to minimize any pain. Then the nurse would push down on my port with her plastic wand. It was essentially like an electrical plug, except the plug part was inside of me and the wall plate/wand would attach to me. It was pain free.

I was hooked up now and ready to go. The nurse left the room and I looked over at John nervously. "I love you."

"I love you too."

I held back my terrified tears once more.

The nurse came back in and informed me that my

numbers were fine and we were ready to proceed.

My first round of chemo was adriamiacin/cytoxin. I was going to be doing that type of chemo for the next four treatments, the next two months of my life, with two more months of another type of chemo to follow. Four months total. I was ready.

She gave me an angel bell to hold and told me to ring the bell if I felt anything different at all. Apparently, some people had allergic reactions to this medicine. You would know relatively quickly if this happened. Mary told me it would take about a half an hour for the drip bag and then she would come back and administer the adriamiacin.

She left and John asked me how I was doing. "Fine." I said. "It didn't hurt at all."

He asked, "Are you okay?"

"Yeah."

Wide-eyed looking at my port he said, "What a trip! This is such a trip!"

It was a trip. The whole thing was so bizarre. Here I was having chemotherapy. John then looked into my eyes and said, "You're so lovely." This was the phrase I cherished hearing from John. I always had. Never did I tire of it. I told him I loved him in return. His love always seemed to make it better. We held hands and chatted a bit. John and I laughed about this and that and then we sat quietly. I realized I was going to be okay.

Sitting through five hours of chemo wasn't going to be so bad. It didn't hurt. I wasn't throwing up or feeling sick in any way. I was fine. After some time passed I told John he could leave and I would call him if I needed him. He questioned again if I was going to be okay if he left. I reassured him I was fine. He helped me get set up, reclined my chair, pulled my book out, set my drink near by me and off he went.

I wasn't ready to talk to anyone else there. They all

looked so sick. I also wasn't ready for questions. Questions would force me to talk and if I talked I would cry. I didn't want to cry in front of people I didn't know, so silent I stayed. I proceeded to read my book.

I did listen in though. The two men in their seventies across from me talked about cures, about insurance, about nutrition, about doctors, and about clinics. Talked or, I should say, complained. Maybe I would complain too if I was seventy having to go through chemo. I don't know.

The women were scattered amongst the men. Most of them were also in their seventies. Like me, they weren't talking either. They didn't look so good. I tried to avoid glancing over at them but I couldn't help but find myself stealing a look or two.

Directly across from me was a younger girl. She had to have been at least ten years younger than me. She looked miserable, not sick mind you, just miserable. Maybe it was the wig she wearing. "Oh God, I don't want to lose my hair!" Her wig was a beautiful long brown full and bouncy wig. Had she had eyebrows, eyelashes and a smile you wouldn't be able to pick her out and identify her as a cancer victim in a line of healthy people. "She was so young. Why so young? That just isn't fair." I thought.

Another woman had spiky short red hair, super sassy just like the woman I encountered months back at my first visit with Dr. Ondreyco. I didn't want to be her. "Damn it! I don't want this. I don't want to do this. I don't want to sit here with all of these sick people. I don't want to lose my hair. I don't want to have some short butch 'I just kicked cancer's ass' haircut. I want my hair. I want this to be over. Just one! Just one!"

Mary came back in and pulled up a chair in front of me. She had a giant plastic syringe with her. It was filled with red liquid that looked like cherry kool-aid. She told me she was going to administer it slowly into my IV and that it would take about thirty minutes or so. She proceeded to inject the colorful cure into my IV. She chatted the entire time telling me about her eight-year-old son, her ex-husband, her divorce, etc.

Thirty minutes later, she was done. Now I just had to sit back and let the next two bags of liquid slowly drip their way through my veins for another three hours. I thanked her and picked up my book again.

Reading kept my mind off of everything. I thought to myself, "This isn't so bad after all. I can get through this. It didn't hurt. I can catch up on reading. Okay, I can do this... Wait, what the heck? My nose hurts. It's a burning feeling. Crap! Do I ring the bell? No. I'm sure it's nothing. Just read. Just one. Crap. It hurts. I wonder if this is a big deal. It's just my nose burning. You're fine Holly. Keep reading."

Right then Mary walked by and I must have had that panicked look in my eye that I get when I'm a little worried. She asked "How you doing Holly?"

"My nose is burning." I replied.

"Oh, that happens to some people. You will just want to take some Aleve and Clariton to relieve that."

There you go. Aleve and Clariton. No big deal. But it did burn. The burning didn't stop. I blocked everything and everyone out and read the rest of the day. I kept looking up at the IV bag halfway gone, three quarters gone. I glanced up at the oversized gaudy clock on the back wall, 2:00, 3:00, 4:00, 4:30 and I was done. I did it. One round of chemo over and done with. One step closer and it wasn't so bad. On the way out one of the nurses told me you'll probably have some mild flu-like symptoms over the weekend. (HA!)

John picked me up and home, sweet, home we went. Our girls were there to greet me when I got home. I relayed to them how it went, what the nurses did, what I did . . . Everything. This was at 4:00 p.m. I made my happy posting on Facebook.

Holly Toner-Rose is happy that chemo

231

was not as scary as she thought it would be.

And as usual Facebook friends were rooting for me.

<u>Matt</u> Excellent News!

<u>Dan</u> Very good news!

I had no idea what I was in for. Taking the nurses' advice I went to the grocery store with Ivy to buy some bland food that I wouldn't mind throwing up. She also recommended not eating any of my favorite foods, because they might not be my favorites anymore if I spent the next week throwing them up. Some soup sounded safe.

By the time I reached the store, nausea was starting to set in. I was unsure what to think at first. "Maybe it will just go away." But it kept getting stronger. "Oh God. I feel sick. Ivy, I don't feel so good." My head started to hurt as well. This was no ordinary headache. This was a tight band going around the back of my head that was getting tighter and tighter, and stronger and stronger. I stared into the aisles, not knowing what I was looking at. I couldn't concentrate. I felt sick, really sick. "Ivy, pick out whatever you want. We need to go baby. Mommy's not feeling so well."

"Okay." she chirped with a smile. She picked out chicken nuggets shaped like dinosaurs and brownies with colored sprinkles on top. That was my Ivy. Innocence. Loveliness.

I made it home and settled into the couch (which was to be my spot for the next four months). I hadn't eaten all day and I needed strength. John went to the kitchen and prepared food for the girls and me. After forcing in a couple of bites, I could eat no more.

Sitting on the couch my head hurt more and more by the minute. The band around the back of my head tightened, and the nausea became more intense. John looked over at me and I wept. "I don't feel good honey."

"Oh, my honey. You have a boo-boo lip." I wept some more. I decided to jump into bed and sleep it all away. I couldn't sleep, though, with nausea that was overwhelming. It felt like I was drunk and spinning, except take away the drunken part, just spinning nausea.

"Make it stop!" And I wept some more. John and the girls came in to try to cheer me up. They all piled in the bed and we watched a movie on John's laptop. I was nestled safely in between my girls and John. I felt sick, but I was safe with my family. One day down.

The next morning, I awoke to the same sickness. I thought to myself, "I'm just going to keep going. I can feel sick all day and lay around or I can feel sick all day and keep going." I was going to keep going.

Picking up the phone I called Leslie to see if they were walking that morning. Ten minutes later I met her and Janeen. I greeted them both with a smile. They, of course, asked how everything went and I told them, "It was the word that was scary. It was just the word 'chemo' that was scary. Once I got there it wasn't so bad. It didn't hurt. I just felt a little sick that's all. Even now, my arm hurts worse than the chemo."

My arm did hurt. In fact it was throbbing. I was still healing from the second surgery just fourteen days earlier. The constant movement of my arm caused by walking was agonizing. I tried to keep my smile up and continue. I thought if I just kept going it would all go away. "Mind over matter. Right?" WRONG!!! My arm hurt. My head hurt. I couldn't concentrate on what Janeen and Leslie were saying. All I heard was "blah blah blah blah," through the throbbing of my head and arm.

Leslie looked over at me and asked how I was doing. Holding back my tears I told her, "not so good." I asked Janeen if I could use her phone to call John. A few minutes later John was there in the car to pick me up. So much for my idea of "I'll just keep going. I can do this. - What was I thinking?" I couldn't do this. I felt like utter crap. And couch bound I went.

233

I had to go back to Dr. Ondreyco's office for my booster shot. This shot was to boost my immune system to prevent me from getting sick on top of chemo. (It was a $3500.00 shot. More than the cost of each chemo. Thank Goodness for insurance). I was in and out of the office in fifteen minutes. Again, the nurse said, "Oh, you'll have some minor flu like symptoms the next couple of days." FLU-LIKE SYMPTOMS MY ASS!

The next few days of chemo for rounds 1, 2, 3 and 4 were as follows. The first symptom, as I mentioned, was the nausea. Surprisingly, this symptom became the least of my worries. Next came the tight band on the back of my head that squeezed harder and harder by the minute causing extreme pain. I can't forget the burning of the nose that lasted for hours at a time. It was the feeling of having diet coke come out of your nose when you laugh - BUT FOR HOURS. No, the Clariton and Aleve did not work. Or maybe they did and what I felt was the mild version.

The next pain that set in was indescribable. The only way I can explain it is that it felt like someone had put my head in a microwave set on high for two minutes. This highly toxic feeling inside my brain was the absolute worst. I think it was this feeling that made me lose all concentration. I wasn't able to do two things at once for months to follow. Cooking and talking to my girls at the same time was too much for me. Driving and talking was near impossible. It was as if my head would explode if I did more than one thing at a time. Chemo must have killed brain cells along with cancer cells. That or my body was using every ounce of energy to keep going under the strains of chemo. Whatever it was, this pain brought me to tears. Then again it might have been the feeling of having two sharp pencils being pushed into the back of my eyes for days on end. This wonderful symptom held me back from reading for months.

Nothing helped any of these symptoms. NOTHING! These were the symptoms on Thursday and Friday. By

Saturday new symptoms set in and don't forget that old ones hadn't left yet. I had the feeling that my skin was black and blue from my ribs up. Just leaning against a pillow felt like it was bruising my skin even more. I'd swear that had I looked in a mirror my skin would have been covered in one dark purple bruise.

There was no day of rest on Sunday. By Sunday my spirits were shot, depression was sinking in and I was an emotional wreck. And to top it off acid-like diarrhea kicked in causing insufferable pain. It left me in tears every hour. I was in the deep dark depths of hell.

But wait! There's more! I also had intense bone pain. My bones felt as if they were decaying from the inside out. The pain was so excruciating.

Monday would come and I would feel the chemo pumping through my heart. I really could. My heart pounded harder and I could feel it pushing the chemo out of my system or at least trying to. This brought on anxiety that I would have a heart attack (one of the chemo precautions - heart failure). I could feel it coming out of my teeth at this point. Sounds crazy, but I did. I also felt it coming out of my esophagus. I would have to take deep breaths, panting, breathing it out. Had there been a color to chemo I would have been breathing fire. This was also the day that depression came on hard and strong. I was usually hysterical at this point. I was battered and beaten.

Tuesday came and I found a glimmer of hope realizing that I was on the last day of my hellish symptoms and I searched deep for my spirit again. Symptoms subsided one by one and I came out of my "chemo coma". I would pick myself up emotionally or I should say John picked me up emotionally.

The only new symptom to appear was the constant drip of my nose. Drip, drip, drip, until the entire inside of my nose was plastered. Out it would come and then drip, drip, drip for days. After Tuesday I would have waves of microwave brain, burning nose and the drip, drip, drip. Wednesday and Thursday a little better.

By the second week after receiving chemo on Friday and Saturday, I felt a little better. Sunday I was hopeful and felt more like me. I was still pretty much exhausted every day by 8:00p.m. That was all the energy my body had to give. On the second Monday after chemo I felt good. I could do this. My spirits picked up. On Tuesday I would be up and about. "I'll go exercise. Yay! I can do this." Wednesday - "Oh God! I don't want to go back. No! I don't want to go back." And every second Thursday - another round of chemo.

And so it went for four months. I think all the nurses were wrong about the mild flu-like symptoms. What they meant to say was "intense hell-like torture chamber symptoms you'll never forget for the rest of your life." That was chemo for me.

After my first round, I really did try my hardest to keep life going. I had tried to go for a walk with Leslie and Janeen - unsuccessful. On Saturday, I tried to clean my house - unsuccessful. Switching one load of laundry left me exhausted and feeling helpless. I broke down crying realizing at this point I wasn't going to be able to do much for months. I was helpless. Now I knew why the genealogist said, "Delegate." I cried in John's arms once more. He told me not to worry. He told me to rest and he would take care of everything. And he did.

My good friend Val was in town during the first round of chemo and everyone was getting together at Katie's.

> Holly Toner-Rose can't wait to see Val
> and everyone at KK's.
>
> Val Me too! Me too! Me too!

I tried to put my mask back on and make a presence at KK's. I lasted about one hour and had to return home. Again, I cried the whole way home and then some.

Most of my day was spent on the couch. I watched rerun after rerun. For days I only ate bits of soup to give my body some strength to fight a little more. I soaked in super hot baths hopeful to alleviate some of my bone pain. Each bath I tried to wash away the depressing thoughts that started pouring out of me. It was getting harder and harder. My last effort to keep up my spirits was walking. I couldn't exercise. I couldn't lift weights. I couldn't run. I couldn't hike, but maybe I could still walk. On the first Monday, five days after my first round, I walked a little and then came home and cried.

Not giving up I tried again on Tuesday. I walked down the sidewalk and tried to hold my head high and fill it with happy thoughts. I grasped for something to be thankful for. I couldn't find anything. Not a thing. I thought about how bad my body felt. How long I had felt bad. How much longer I had to go. Tears started pouring out of me as I walked on. "God, I can't do this. I don't have the strength to do this. Help me! Help me! I'm not strong enough for this. I can't do this. Please God help me." I was losing the fight. Cancer was winning.

I made my way home and made a beeline to John. I collapsed into his lap sobbing like a five year old. "Oooooh boobakins. My little bilikin" he poured out to me as he stroked my hair.

"I can't do this John. It's killing my spirit. It's killing my body AND my spirit. It's not fair. It's not fair," I cried out.

John reassured me, "I'm sorry honey. You're doing so good. You've already gotten through one round. That's one less you have to do. You can do it."

I sobbed and sobbed into his chest, "I can't! I can't! I'm not strong enough for this. I can't do it this anymore. I still have seven more rounds to go. I can't do three and a half more months of this. I can't!" He held me tight in his arms, like a child. I don't know what I would have done without him. His strength carried me through every moment like this and I had so many of them in the months to follow.

With John's help I found renewed strength and I wasn't ready to give up the fight. Mediation was my new approach. I sat outside on my quilted blanket in the shady grass and stretched and breathed in the fresh open air trying to push out the toxins and tears from my tattered body.

I looked up at the sky above me and I prayed and pleaded once more. "Please God, help me get through this. I don't think I can do this one alone God. I need you. Please help me, Jesus. Please help me." Tears streaked my cheeks again. I battled to find my spirit again all day. I felt defeated.

The next morning as I walked on I glanced up the sky reflecting back over the past week. I was starting to feel better. I made it. I did it. Yesterday later in the day some of symptoms had started to subside. God did hear me and came to my rescue. I had him on my side giving my strength. I could do this. I could. "Thank you God."

Chapter Twenty-One

April 1st. April Fool's Day. Sick or not sick I couldn't let the day go by without doing something. I had always been a fan of April Fool's Day. Once in college, my friend Val and I woke up super early with a stack a signs we had made the night before. We went to each and every shower on all four floors of our dorm, entered the shower stall, turned on the water, closed and locked the door, posted a sign inside "April Fool's Day!", and then crawled underneath the door leaving it locked to present the appearance that it was occupied. We watched girl after girl toting her basket of toiletries to shower for the day and each girl angrily returning with dry hair. We heard talk about it all over campus. I know, not very green of us, but this was back in the 1980's. No one thought about their footprint on the Earth or the water we were wasting. We were eighteen and only thought about the laughter we had just shared.

Every year I schemed up something fun. So, being a fan of this holiday I couldn't let it pass me by. I posted on Facebook:

> Holly Toner-Rose "OPRAH CALLED BACK!!!!!!! CHICAGO HERE I COME!!!!!! I'M GONNA BE ON THE OPRAH SHOW!!!!!!

An incredible number of responses came in on Facebook and phone calls by the dozen. Everyone wanted to know when I was going to be on the show, were they flying me out, who was going with, could they come with, etc. I couldn't believe people actually fell for it. It was April Fool's Day!

Later that day as I worked on my book doing edits a nagging feeling lingered that I was "supposed to" do something with my book. This thought energized me.

As young as age five I recall writing stories. I clearly

remember sitting at the desk I made out of purple paisley storage boxes stacked on top of each other pouring out my creative thoughts. I filled my kitty notebooks. Thinking each and every line was brilliant. I dreamed of growing up to become an author. Looking back through them now, not a one was good.

I'm not sure what happened or why, but I stopped writing at some point. Never in my wildest dreams did I think I would yearn to write again. In college I envied every piece written by Val, my college roommate, who went on to become an accomplished singer/songwriter in the band Loretta Lynch. (If you are looking for a little bit of front porch, a little bit back woods, a little tear in your beer, a little knife in your back...then Loretta Lynch is for you. Please check out her music at www.lorettalynch.com) In college we all knew she would succeed in her music. She is soooo talented. Her words captured you every time. I did not possess her talent, but I was forced to write anyway.

I do remember that once I was called in for a meeting with my English professor. My first thought was "Crap! My essay was that bad, he needs to have a meeting with me!" As I sat waiting for the negative criticism, the opposite happened. He accused me of plagiarizing. He thought it was written so well that it could not have been mine. My startled look must have shocked him into realizing that I did indeed write it myself. I'm not sure if every other piece I wrote in his class was awful and I deserved the accusation or maybe he was a great teacher and my writing skills improved over the semester.

At any rate, here I was, some twenty years later with a book in my hand. I was starting to think about the real possibility that I could publish it. People seemed to like it, although maybe I was just receiving positive responses due to the fact that I was a cancer patient. Who was going to tell me they didn't like it?

I began creating a cover for my book in my mind. I wanted the cover to represent me, who I was, my spirit. I wanted my girls to see me in it, in case I wasn't there and they didn't remember me. I wanted them to be proud of me - proud of their mommy.

My favorite piece of artwork is one by Lichtenstein. Every time I look at the print, it puts a smile on face. It brings on a carefree and youthful feeling and fills me with enthusiasm and optimism. The painting reflected how I felt about life. Life was something to appreciate and enjoy! To be happy - No matter what life threw at you, be it a ball or cancer, you can't stop enjoying life. I believe you have a choice to smile and throw the ball back or drop the ball jumping out of the game. I was going to keep playing the game. That was how I felt. I wanted to share that feeling inside me.

I couldn't use Lichtenstein's painting on my cover, so I thought what if I changed it some. That is what he had done too, altering a travel ad. What if I made the girl me? It was my story, my feelings, my reflection . . . It also symbolized my journey through breast cancer. The ball was cancer that was thrown in my direction. I found a way to pull something beautiful out of cancer. I was able to open my eyes and see the beauty in it - I saw all of the wonderful people surrounding me holding me up. I saw humanity flourish. I saw love in the eyes of my family. I could garner that happy feeling and throw that ball right back with everyone supporting me.

As I thought about these feelings, I thought about my girls. "I don't want to die. I want to be around for them. I want them to know who I am through me, not some picture that I try to capture my spirit in. I love them!!!

With a picture in my mind I then thought about who could pull it off. A few years back, John's friend Kenny Richardson painted a picture of John for a collection he was creating, and he was able to capture John's spirit. I thought he might be able to do the same for me. Having known us for years he knew a little about who I was.

I knew this wasn't his style - Lichtenstein's famous pop art with the dot application, but I trusted he could transfer my essence on to a canvas. I phoned him and asked him if he could do my book cover and explained what I wanted. He said he would be honored. (Now, that I believe I'm going to be okay I must admit I'm a bit embarrassed. It's a picture of me. Not only did I think it would make a great book cover I decided to use it for our non-profit as our logo for our "Don't be a Chump! Check for a Lump!" campaign. Please remember I thought I was dying. John told me, "Holly you have immortalized yourself." I almost have to giggle when we sell our t-shirts. I want to jokingly say, "Would anyone like to buy a t-shirt of me? Anyone? Did anyone NOT get a t-shirt of me?" What can I do but laugh about it now?)

Later that afternoon I had my appointment with Dr. Zannis. He wanted to make sure I was healing properly. I told John I was okay for this one by myself and besides, who could give you bad news on April Fool's Day? There was no possibility of bad news today.

Wanting Dr. Zannis to hear all of my praises for him, I brought with me a copy of my book for him to read (Now I wished I had waited to give him the edited version instead of my painkiller-induced copy. Oh well). I also wrote him a card thanking him, essentially for my life. He had treated me with such care and kindness. Words could not express how thankful we were to have him as my doctor.

In his office, he checked my progress and informed me that I was healing just fine. He graciously accepted my book to read and my card.

While in the office he asked me how chemo was going. Putting on my happy shield I told him I was doing okay. He asked if I was going to cut my hair. He must have witnessed time after time how hard it was for women to lose their hair. I made a mental note to hurry and cut my hair. I knew I only had a matter of days left.

Thursday, April 2ⁿᵈ, 2009. My appointment with my oncologist's P.A. was scheduled for the day. They wanted an update on how I was surviving chemo and if I needed any medication or had any problems. Patiently I sat. Bill, the P.A., sauntered in casually and sat down with my four-inch chart in hand. "So how did it go?"

I wanted to respond with, "How do you think? You idiot. I just did a round of chemo a week ago. It was the worst experience of my entire life and I have to do it seven more times!"

Instead I replied with, "Good."

"Any complications?"

Again, I wanted to shout, "Are you kidding me? Do you call microwave brain, intense bone pain and acid-like diarrhea, complications!!!!"

I calmly replied, "No". He ran through a few of the symptoms that I might be experiencing and I answered, "Yes." "Yes." "Yes".

Quickly, he performed a check on my vitals and nonchalantly told me, "Well, the good news is whatever you experienced this round is pretty much what you can expect for the rest of chemo."

"So it isn't accumulative?"

"No. The symptoms you had this past week will most likely be the symptoms every time." He then asked, "Are you going to cut your hair?"

I thought to myself, "Again with the hair. Damn! I better hurry."

"When will it fall out?"

"You have about two weeks from the date of your first treatment." That meant I had less than a week to go. I left convincing myself that I had great news. Now I knew what to expect for the next three and a half months. It wasn't going to get any worse.

Every day I was filled with dread over losing my hair. I was going to be bald. I knew I should focus on the fact that I was going to be okay. Hair was just a part of vanity. It wasn't me – or was it?

Red hair was a part of my identity. Growing up with red hair I was one of the three little red-heads (my sisters all have red hair too). In grade school I was the token redheaded girl and was called "carrot top" among other things. In high school it progressed to just "red." Once I recall cruising down Central, a local pastime on Friday and Saturday nights back in the day, with the top to my MG down. My car started to overheat and some guy with a loud speaker attached to his car called out, "Hey Red! Your car is on fire." And then the moment I met John when he called out, "A red-head." Red hair was a part of me and who I was.

Sharon, a survivor herself, had emailed me that day confirming my hair would start to fall out fifteen days after my first treatment. I cried all day about my hair. I lay in bed with tears streaming down. Hannah, Ivy and John all tried to cheer me up but nothing worked. "I don't waaant to lose my hair. I don't waaaant to be bald. It's not fair!" My whining continued all day long like this. I didn't even care that Hannah and Ivy saw me crying. Normally I would have hid all of these fears and tears from them. I didn't care right now though. I was going to be bald in a few days. It wasn't fair so I cried and cried some more.

Hannah, always sympathetic to someone's tears, tried again and again to cheer me up. As I was lying on the bed whining she came in with a smile and said "Mommy, why don't you just paint your world purple? Get happy purple shoes and a purple shirt and a purple purse. Paint your whole world purple, Mommy." I sure did love her. She knew I loved purple and that the color always made me happy. She was so beautiful to think about that.

That is exactly what I did that day. I bought patent

leather purple shoes, a matching purple purse and a lavender blouse. I was going to paint my world purple just like Hannah advised. I wasn't going to have hair in a couple of days but I had Hannah to help me paint my world purple. What more did I really need in life?

I wasn't going to be mad any longer. I had to let it go. I had to let my hair go. Damn it!

> <u>Holly Toner-Rose</u> is thinking that life is
> too short to be mad about the little things.
> Be happy! Damn it!

The next evening, John and I had plans to go to his cousin Kari's wedding. John wasn't sure he wanted to go, but I did. I wanted to go be social. I wanted to chat and laugh and dance. I wanted to live. I was also well aware of the fact that I didn't have too many opportunities ahead of me with hair.

As I got ready for my last evening out with hair I asked the girls "Hair straight or curly?"

"CURLY!"

So, curly it was.

I donned my new pretty purple shoes and pretty purple purse. John and I were late and missed the actual wedding. While we waited for the wedding party to make their grand entrance we mingled with all of his family. They all asked how I was doing. I responded to each one that I was doing fine. I told them all it wasn't so bad (Lie).

The wedding party entered and we sat down at a table with all of John's siblings. Round the table we went. How are you? Great! You? How are the kids? Great! Yours? Etc. All I could really think about was "I'm going to be bald in a couple of days. BALD! Don't cry Holly. Just one! Just one!"

After dinner, microwave head started to set in, wave upon wave. Each one getting stronger. I was trying to ignore it hoping it would end soon. John looked over at me and noticed I wasn't doing so well. He asked me if I wanted to leave. I pleaded, "No." He took my hand and led me outside to get a breath of fresh air. I felt like Cinderella and the clock had struck twelve (8:00 p.m. for me). I wasn't going to turn into a pumpkin but my body was going to shut down on me.

After a while we went back inside. I asked John if we could wait until after the wedding couple had their first dance so we could enjoy one dance together. One dance with my husband was all I wanted. Toasts were made and of all the women cried. I'm not sure if I was crying with sentiment towards the newlywed couple or crying for me and my hair. I think a little of both.

The father of the bride then stood up and made a toast. I thought about John toasting Hannah and Ivy on their wedding days. I thought about the tears he would shed on those days. I thought about how beautiful our girls would look at their weddings. I then thought, "Oh God, I don't want to miss their weddings. I want to be there. I want to hold their little faces and kiss their foreheads and tell them I love them and watch them, nervous and giddy, enter into the beautiful gift of marriage. Please let me be there. Hair or no hair, I want to be there."

A few toasts and a few dances later everyone was asked to join in. John took my hand and led me to the dance floor. My head was killing me, but I didn't care. My honey had me in his arms now and I was okay. Again, I fought back my tears. I loved him so much.

The song ended and I was ready to go home now. I had my dance in with my hubby and I really, really didn't feel well. As we walked off the dance floor the B-52's came on. Pre-chemo days we would have happily jumped back onto the dance floor with a shimmy of our own, but not today. Life had changed so much. I couldn't do the same things. I was missing out on life. Chemo was killing me.

Sunday, April 5th, 2009. It was my last day with hair. John's brother Stephen was coming over that evening to take family pictures for us. As I was getting ready I started to get a little anxious. It was getting later and later and John hadn't heard from Stephen. If we missed the sunset we would have to wait until the next day. Stephen didn't realize how important this was to me. I'm sure he thought if he was too late there was always tomorrow - always another sunset. But there wasn't always tomorrow. Tomorrow the sunset would be there but my hair might not be. Tomorrow I may be bald. John didn't seem to care either. No one realized how important this was to me, except me. I was really the only one living through each moment of this. No one but me would feel how crappy chemo was, how agonizing microwave brain was, how awful it was to think about being bald . . . No one but me.

Tears started to well up again and my make-up was starting to smear, which made me cry even more. I cried to John. "Everything is going to be fine Holly. He's going to be here. Just stop worrying." John reassured me. I didn't believe him.

At that point I called Leslie. "I have a Wine emergency! Can you please bring me a glass of wine? I'm starting to freak out and we're supposed to take pictures and now I'm crying. I just need to chill." She showed up at my door minutes later with a smile and a bottle of wine. She was always so kind. She listened and helped calm me down. She never hesitated when a friend was in need.

Stephen did show up on time (sorry Stephen). We walked over to the country club to take pictures on the golf course. He must have taken a hundred pictures - Pictures of our whole family, pictures of the girls and me, pictures of John and me, and pictures of the girls. They were the last pictures of me with hair.

That was what I had been waiting for. Now was the time. I took a look at myself in the mirror and gave myself a pep talk. "I can do this! I can do this! I'm ready!" I put my hair in a low ponytail in the back, grabbed my sewing scissors off of my vanity and called for John. I asked him to cut it off for me.

"Holly, just wait for it to fall out. I wouldn't cut it." I couldn't wait anymore. I couldn't wake up day after day and wonder if this was going to be the day my hair would fall out. Would this be the day? Would this be the day? I wanted it gone. No more worries, no more waiting, no more.

I reached behind me with courage and gripped my ponytail tight. I started sawing away strand by strand, chunk by chunk. I was doing it. I was cutting my hair off. And voila! I did it. I looked again in the mirror. "Okay. I don't look so bad. That wasn't so bad. I did it! I did it!" Proudly I held up my ponytail high in my hand and John took a picture of me. John told me how great I looked. I was okay. One step down.

An hour later I did show up at Leslie's door. When she opened the door I held up my ponytail and exclaimed "Hair emergency!" She helped me trim up the back so it didn't look like I took a butcher knife to my hair. We sat at her kitchen bar chatting and her husband Todd walked in the door.

Leslie cried out in excitement, "Look at Holly's hair!" trying to cheer me on. Todd didn't exactly give the response either one of us was looking for.

Todd looked confused and blurted out, "Why did you do that?" He also wasn't thinking I was going to be bald in a day or two. In Todd's defense most men responded this way. I didn't really care though. I made it through step number one. Now I had step number two ahead of me.

Holly Toner-Rose IS TAKING IT ONE STEP AT A TIME.

248

Chapter Twenty-Two

Our family was holding up pretty well considering. John was my hero and the girls were my heroines. They all kept their fears from me. I was so thankful. John never revealed his fears. Ivy never wanted to think about it or talk about it. "Hear no evil, See no evil" was her motto. Hannah, on the other hand, thought about the "what ifs?" the future, the possibilities . . . She was also very strong. She didn't want me to be upset by her emotions, so she hid them. The two months were too much for my beautiful little eleven year-old. She had so many emotions that needed to come out, and come out they did.

The next day, my family came over to celebrate my dad's and my sister Sheree's birthdays. Hannah and Ivy had made them cards earlier in the day.

Hannah's cards were a special treat to receive. She always put so much thought into each and every one. She considered the person and their likes and created her card with their personality in mind. Her past cards included a pop-up card with Grandpa shooting a bear, an actual record decorated for her daddy and, of course, purple cards with pictures of her for mommy. We all adored her cards.

That evening, as we were leaving the house, Hannah frantically ran about. Her card for Grandpa was not finished yet. I hurried her along, trying to get her out the door. She was upset that her masterpiece was not finished. I reassured her it was okay and that he would love it anyway. Hannah was not budging. She wanted to finish her card. I was anxious with Grandma and Grandpa in the car ready to go and I sternly told her, "Hannah we are going now." She huffed and puffed. I started to raise my voice. "Hannah, we have to go now. Forget the card. Finish it later. We have to go!" She still didn't budge. "Hannah, if you don't go now Kelly can not sleepover this

Friday." I knew it was a mistake to say before the words even left my mouth. This was not one of my "good Mommy moments".

Whenever I threw out a consequence I had to keep to it. It was one of my parenting rules. Stick by what you say. I regretted threatening her with a punishment. She just wanted her gift to be as nice as possible.

I was in a losing battle at this point. Once I angered her, she needed time to forgive and forget (She was like me). John was always more successful than me in pulling her out of an angry tornado but, then again, he was used to dealing with me. He knew all the tricks after seventeen years of handling me with care. Hannah slowly inched her way out of the house, eyes glaring deep into my soul. She wasn't going to let this one go.

We went to dinner and enjoyed the evening with little interruptions. The next day, though, everything came out. Hannah asked again about Kelly staying over. I told her I had to stick with my original punishment. Looking back I should have made an exception to my rule. I was wrong.

Hannah screamed when she heard my refusal and ran to her room, slamming the door behind her. I barged into her room and yelled out, "Do NOT slam this door again!" She shrieked once more. I left the room and next I heard a loud bang. My emotions were out of control and instead of taking time to calm down to figure out the right thing to do I marched right back in. "HANNAH, What did you do?" I turned towards her door and saw a big gaping hole in her door. "OH MY GOSH, HANNAH! YOU CANNOT DESTROY PROPERTY! You are going to have to go to the bank and take out your savings and have Daddy take to you to Home Depot to buy a new door. YOU CANNOT BREAK STUFF!

She screamed back, "Aaaaaaaaaahhhhh! Get out! Get out!!!!!!"

John came in at that point, "WHAT IS GOING ON?"

"She broke her door! Just look at it! She broke her door!"

"Well, she can hang a poster over it."

"Are you kidding me? She broke it. She needs to pay for it."

John and I fought for the next two hours over the consequences. My idea was cancer or no cancer in our family there were boundaries that you had to uphold. John thought she deserved a break and she needed to get out all of her emotions and anger. I disagreed vehemently and so did he. We went to sleep with no exchanges of kisses or words. Anger filled the room. I prayed to God for wisdom and strength and then cried myself to sleep.

Wednesday, April 8th. We woke to the same anger. I had my first meeting with Dr. Quiet that day. Still angry, I passed on his offer to come with me. This was just a get-to-know the doctor and what was to come meeting.

When she walked in and greeted me I instantly knew why Dr. Zannis had referred me to her. She was the female version of him. She was compassionate and caring. She sat and talked with me, not to me, for an hour. She asked how I was getting through it, how my husband and I were getting through it, and how my girls were getting through it. I must have shown my fears in my eyes.

She told me "Most young women who go through breast cancer have a hard time with their children. The children are scared and don't know how to deal with their emotions. They will test all of their boundaries right now. They want to know that nothing has changed and they are still safe. You need to keep up the discipline and every boundary in place." As she was telling me all of this, I thought of Hannah and her punching a hole through the door. She was so scared. My poor baby. I was so thankful for this doctor in front of me. God had placed this wonderful woman in front of me, counseling me on how to help our girls. I needed help and God provided it.

I cried to Dr. Quiet, "Thank you so much. You just explained my oldest daughter." I proceeded to tell her about our experience the night before. She counseled me some more and I was thankful. She advised me to keep trying to get our girls to talk about it. Persuade them to let their fears out.

Before leaving she also told me to be careful and said that most women gained twenty pounds during chemo. "Was she kidding me? Not only do I have to go through chemo, lose my hair and my parenting skills, I have to get fat on top of it." I wasn't going to let that happen.

When I left her office I felt much better about Hannah. I immediately called John to relay what Dr. Quiet had passed on to me about keeping boundaries up, etc. Our conversation was quick. I think we needed to vent ourselves. Maybe we should have broken a few doors to let out our steam as well.

Later that day I planned to take Ivy and Hannah to Taliesin, Frank Lloyd Wright's home in Scottsdale, Az. Ivy was doing a report on him and I had promised to take her on the Taliesin tour. Round two of chemo was scheduled for the next day so I knew I would be out of commission for a week. Today was my last remaining free day.

On our way to Taliesin I tried to draw out the girls emotions. First I reassured them that I was going to be okay and then explained to them how I was feeling and how I thought they might be feeling. I asked them to share their thoughts with me. I started to say, "I know our situation . . ."

And Hannah abruptly cut me off and interjected, "Is Intense!"

"Yes, it is intense Hannah. And unfair. Unfair for all of us. You both are so young to have to deal with this kind of stress. We don't have a choice though. This is what God handed us, for whatever reason, and we have to deal with it. We are just going to have to get through it."

I then went through the range of emotions I thought they must be feeling and appropriate responses. I told them,

"It's okay to be mad and angry and scared, but it's not okay to break doors or hit people or hurt yourself. Sick or not sick it is not acceptable. You can beat your pillow and your stuffed animals, you can cry, and you can scream, but you can't break things or hurt yourself." Hannah eyes were glazed and fixated out the window as every word breezed by her. She was getting madder by the minute.

Ivy jumped in saying, "Can we stop talking about it now?" They had listened to enough of my advice and lecture.

When we arrived at Taliesin Ivy and me were ready for fun. Hannah was still brooding over our conversation in the car. I decided to just let her be. There was no sense in trying to force her to be happy. That backfired every time with her. As we proceeded through the tour, I noticed Hannah's blue eyes brighten at every turn. She soaked up and admired the essence of Frank Lloyd Wright.

At the end of the tour I asked them both if they would like to go to the Taliesin School of Architecture. Ivy jumped in and said "Yeah!" Hannah was silent.

I knew she wanted to scream out with excitement to me, "Mom, that was so cool. I loved every room. Did you see this... and this... and this ... But she was still mad at me and wasn't able to voice a word.

Hannah had always been like that. She was like me in that way. I took my own sweet time forgiving someone if they hurt my feelings or made me mad, right or wrong. I was going to make them pay for hurting me. We shared this spiteful trait.

I recalled one memorable instance with Hannah. For years I drove the girls to school and we passed by the same gas station every day. Hannah commented that no one was ever there and they would probably go out of business in the near future. Day after day, she mentioned the station and her prediction while we were stopped at the red light.

Hannah awoke one school morning as mad as she could be. Every step in getting her ready for school was like pulling hair. I tried to usher her out the door but her shoes didn't match her outfit. (This was back in her matching days.) If she was wearing a red shirt, she had to be wearing red shoes, blue shirt-blue shoes. This made it difficult every morning since I could not afford to buy a pair of shoes in every color for her and could not for the life of me convince her that blue tennis shoes did match a red shirt. (THEY MATCHED EVERYTHING!!!)

We finally made it out the door after I screamed and hollered at her. I was given the silence treatment the entire drive to school as my punishment for raising my voice. And then we pulled up to the light, that very same light we sat at day after day, but today the gas station on the corner was gone. Overnight it had been bulldozed. All that was left was a large dirt lot and chain link fence bordering it. I gasped and said, "Hannah! Look, it's gone. They finally tore it down. You were right!" She said nothing. She was still mad at me.

I knew inside her voice was screaming out, "Mom! Look! Mom! They tore it down just like I said. Look!" Anger silenced her excitement then as it had silenced her at Taliesin. She was dying to tell me how much she loved it but couldn't. I knew though. She didn't have to tell me. I knew. That's what moms do.

That night at dinner I asked them again about Taliesin and their favorite parts of the tour. Ivy said she would love to go to the Taliesin School, and with that response all of Hannah's pent up fears and anger came bursting out. She screamed, "YOU DON'T EVEN WANT TO BE AN ARCHITECT, YOU NEVER HAVE!!!!! YOU'VE HEARD ME SAY I WANT TO BE AN ARCHITECT LIKE A MILLION TIMES. AND NOW YOU WANT TO, WELL YOU CAN'T!!!!"

My poor little girl. She must have had so many fears bottled up that she couldn't share with me or anyone else. Her and Ivy both. They were so strong through all of it. I'm so proud of how they carried themselves through everything. I love them both so much.

That night I cried again. I prayed to God to give me strength, to help me and our children and John get through this - somehow. John held me in his arms as I dozed off to sleep.

Chapter Twenty-Three

Thursday, April 9th, 2009. Chemo round number two. I was scared. I didn't want to go back and enter hell once again. I didn't want more of that awful venom inside of me.

Sitting on my bedroom floor I cried out my fears and a whole lot of tears. "I don't want to go. I don't want to go back! I just started to live life again. I don't want to go!!! Why me? Why me? I can't do this. How am I going to get through seven more rounds of this? SEVEN! Oh God, Why? I don't want to go back!!!! I don't want to go!!!!!"

Finally, all cried out, I picked myself up and went to find John. As I walked past our front door, which is next to our bedroom, I noticed the door was slightly open. As I went to close the door, something caught me eye. Someone had come by and left me a bright bouquet of flowers to light up my day. There was no card, no note – just pretty flowers.

My mind raced to the minutes before. Whoever came to the door must have heard me crying and decided not to knock. "How embarrassing! Who cares! I have to go to chemo today. Whoever it was, they would be crying too, if they were me."

A smile appeared as I peered at my pretty bouquet. My fears lifted and my spirit grew. People were so caring and kind. I was so lucky.

> Holly Toner-Rose is loving the flowers that showed up on her doorstep today. Thank you, whoever you are! They brightened my day.

John drove me to my chemo appointment. I held his hand tightly trying to gather his strength. I needed every bit of it. When we arrived, I kissed him goodbye, and told him I would call when I was done. I stood tall, took a deep breath, told my myself I was going to be okay and made my way to the dusty pink Lazy Boy chair for one more round. Same procedure. . . Easy chair, IV, laptop, sick people surrounding me, burning in my nose, heart pumping, self distraction, "Just one!".

Five hours later, one more round - done. I called Katie on the way home. She was always wonderful. "Congratulations! You are half way to half way!!!!"

Katie is so positive. She put a smile on my face and made me laugh for ten straight months. I'm so thankful she's my friend. Katie was one of the few people I took calls from while in my "chemo coma". She always cheered me up. I tried my best not to cry to her. Again, I didn't want anyone to feel sorry for me. But, on many occasion I did cry and she listened and then she made me laugh somehow or another. I love her.

Everyone else who phoned during the first five days after a chemo injection was told to call me back on Tuesday. Tuesday was the last day of my chemo coma and I was usually coming out of my depression by then. Sheree called me every single Tuesday after chemo. She'd cheerily say, "It's Tuesday. You said I could call." Julie would call. Leslie would call and see if I wanted to try to get out to walk. My mom would call, Shelley, Alisha, Carol, Brenda. . . Etc.

I had so many wonderful people helping me out each round. Brenda and Alisha arrived every week to clean my house. They were never bare handed either. They brought soup and movies and cards and books. Ruth and Katie showed up my doorstep with yellow gloves on ready to scrub my floors and more. Lorie routinely came by every Monday night to prepare dinner for us. It didn't matter that I was never up for conversation. I was still down on Mondays but she was always there. John's mom in town from Utah came over and washed twenty loads of laundry and folded them with love. Everyone reached out to help us in one way or another. I truly feel blessed to have so many beautiful people around us.

Easter came and went during that round of chemo. The

257

girls went to Mark and Teryle's house to spend the day with John's family and all of the cousins. John stayed by my side. The girls returned that evening with cousin Miah in tow, ready for a sleepover. I didn't mind at all. I wanted them all near me, even if I was sick.

Monday, April 13th, 2009. Thirteen - Never a good day. I woke up to a house full of giggling girls. I still wasn't feeling up to par, but then again I never was anymore. Proceeding to get ready, I jumped in the shower like any other day. I put shampoo in my hair and started to massage it into my scalp. What happened next was horrifying. I pulled my hands away from my head only to find them covered in hair. Not just a little hair, mind you, but completed covered. "Oh my gosh! Oh my gosh! It's happening! It's really happening! I don't want to be bald. I don't want to be bald." The shower did little to wash away my fears. Now I had more tears flowing down my face than water. I ran my fingers through my hair again and again. I tried to rid myself of the strands dangling, but they just kept coming. More and more and more and more. "I don't want to be bald. Why me? WHY ME? THIS ISN'T FAIR! I DON'T WANT TO BE BALD!"

After my cry-fest in the shower I continued to get ready. I stood before the mirror brushing out my hair. Large piles came out with each stroke. I threw the brush down. "I just won't touch my hair anymore. Maybe it will stay in for a little bit longer." Right then I heard the doorbell ring. John's brother Danny had arrived to pick up his daughter Miah. Quickly, I wiped away my tears and went to the door and I tried to greet him with a smile. He asked how I was doing. Immediately I cried out, "My hair is falling out."

"Is it falling out slowly?" he asked.

"NO!" With my fingers spread out, I put both hands through my hair to show him the large clumps that would follow. "It just keeps coming and coming. It's all falling out. I don't want to be bald!" I whimpered.

"I'm sorry Holly." He tried to comfort me but it did no

good. I was going to be bald. I cried most of that day grieving for me and my hair. I made my pathetic posting on Facebook.

> <u>Holly Toner-Rose</u> is trying really hard to remember that she gets to live a long happy life, she said while pulling out huge chunks of hair. Waaahhhh!!! I don't want to be bald.

Of course, people responded with warm and wonderful thoughts.

> <u>Victoria</u> I have a medium blonde wig. Would you like to borrow as needed. You could even use it now. Just tuck the hair you have under it. Let me know.

> <u>Valerie</u> You are and will continue to be beautiful, no matter what! But I'm sorry that you have to go through this, and don't blame you for feeling the way you do. You are so loved, my friend!

> <u>Teri</u> My Aunt Mary lost her hair going through the same thing and it came back thicker, shinier and no gray! Strange silver lining, no? Best of luck to you Holly!

> <u>Leslie</u> Hair, schmair! It's overrated!! We just care about YOU!

> <u>Vicki</u> As we say in our household: Bald is Beautiful! You're my hero for going through this with such a great sense of humor.

> <u>Jennifer</u> I have other friends going thru this now too. Seeing those clumps of hair coming out is the hardest part for everyone it seems. Have a good cry, get a little mad, and then think how gorgeous you'll be in wigs. Thinking of you. And

am sooo sorry you have to deal with this. Good thing you're gorgeous no matter what!!!

Alisha Holly, you radiate beauty from the inside out. Hair or no hair; you are beautiful!

Anita You get to live a wonderful long and happy life and you hair will be back in no time, better than ever. If I can do anything.... I am here! But I am sorry for your loss... you are pretty no matter what!

Eric Since my color is closest to yours I can give you mine if you like.

Lorraine Well, at least you can now change your hair color and length with your mood. Just like a Chrissy doll. :) Let me know if you need anything, sis.

Holly Toner-Rose I'm putting on my wig and a smile. Thanks for the cheers everyone. I needed them!

I wish I could say all of the beautiful blessings and humorous comments took my tears away, but they didn't. My hair was coming out, beautiful blessings or not, I was going to be bald.

The next day I had an early appointment to have my blood checked. Dr. Ondreyco had me scheduled every three weeks for check-ups. I jumped in the shower. Again, clump after clump after clump streamed down. While dressing I tried to block out the thought of being bald. I tried to push it far, far away. I applied my makeup hoping maybe I could make myself feel pretty. It didn't work.

I picked up the blow dryer and turned in on. As the hot wind blew in my face, strands of hair flew by me. I pulled down on my hair with my big round brush like I had every day for years and I saw the roots on the end of my hair being pulled down with it. More and more and more hair. I emptied my brush and started again. More and more and more hair. What was I to do? "OH MY GOD. WHAT DO I DO? WHAT DO I DO?" I stood there running my fingers through my hair again. Each time my fingers were tangled in piles of red hair. This was too much for me. "I can't do this!!! I CAN'T DO THIS!" I ran and grabbed some scissors. I ran back to the mirror with scissors in hand. GET THIS OFF OF ME. GET IT OFF." I sobbed. I chopped away at my hair, hacking large chunks at a time. It was a "Mommy Dearest" clip if I ever saw one. "GET IT OFF OF ME." "JOHN!!! JOHN!!! HELP ME, JOHN!!! GET IT OFF!!! GET IT OFF!!! GET THE CLIPPERS!! JUST GET IT OFF!!" (As I write this down I'm sobbing reliving it.)

John ran and found the clippers he used on his hair on occasion. Good ol' barber style clippers. He calmed me down a bit and reassured me it was going to be okay. "It's just hair. It will grow back. I bet you look good with short hair." He buzzed away and a few minutes later all of my hair was one inch long.

"I look like a boy. I look ugly!" I cried.

"No you don't. You look punk rock honey. You look lovely." I wept some more in his arms.

Emotionally defeated I wiped my tears away, left John's office and sulked back to my room to finish getting ready. I stood looking at myself in the mirror. "So, this is me now. Me with really short ugly hair. I'm ugly." and I sobbed some more. Back to the closet I went to cry my heart out. I cried every last drop I had in me that day. !" I cried for being ugly. I cried for having to go do chemo. I cried for still being in pain from surgery. I cried for getting cancer. I cried Why Me?????

After a while, there were no more tears to weep so I picked myself up. I couldn't cry forever. Thinking that if I put on something pretty it might elevate my mood, I flipped through my closet looking for any of my back-up outfits that always looked good on.

Popping out at me was a dainty royal blue sundress with peasant style stitching around the bottom. I smiled at the thought, "Blue always looks good on me. Maybe I can just accentuate my eyes and no one will pay attention to my hair." I slipped the dress on and stood in front of the mirror again. "Not bad I guess. If I had to have super short hair I guess I look okay.

Looking for approval I walked back into John's office. I stood before him with my toes turned in and clutching my fingers, they way I always did when I was nervous and scared. He still looked at me with a twinkle in his eye. He didn't care about my hair. He loved me. I love him so.

> <u>Holly Toner-Rose</u> wants to say, "My hubby is my hero!"

I wasn't exactly ready to brave the world with my new haircut. John loved me regardless of hair but the world wouldn't. Needing to still feel like myself, I put on the wig that made me feel most like Holly. Wearing the long red wig, I stood in front of the entryway mirror pulling it this way and that. I hated it. It was all poufy - not me. It wasn't my hair. I wanted my hair back.

"You ready?" John asked with a confused look. "I don't know why you just don't go without the wig? You look great without it."

"I look ugly. And I hate this wig. I don't want to wear wigs! I want MY hair." I grumbled for another few minutes.

We went to the doctor and when I came home I wrote "Day one with a wig" and posted it on facebook. I also changed my profile picture to the new me with a buzz.

> <u>Day one with a wig!</u>
>
> Wednesday, April 15, 2009 at 11:38am |
>
> I had to go to the doctor's office yesterday.

My hair was coming out by the handful so I figured it was time to shave it off. I couldn't have my red hair flying about in public. John broke out the trimmers and gave me an Avengers buzz cut. (I look very punk rock!) Afterwards, I had to get to the doctor's office. I wasn't feeling well at all physically, or emotionally. I quickly put on my new wig, looked in the mirror, and I was not happy with what I saw. It was not me. It was a wig, not my hair. There was nothing I could do, so off we went to the doctor.

While in the waiting room, I was feeling physically ill. I thought I was going to vomit and my head felt like it had been stuffed into a microwave for a few minutes. I saw the old woman, with really bad hair, across from me looking at me sympathetically. I knew my face was showing my physical agony. She kept giving me kind looks while waiting. I was finally called in to the doctor, they took some blood, and back home we went.

When we walked in the doorway I looked again at myself in the hall mirror. I then realized I had put my wig on wrong. I practically put it on sideways. My hair was worse than the old lady in the waiting room. John said "No wonder that lady was looking at you sympathetically." John and I just thought I looked really bad in wigs before we left.

I did figure out how to properly place a wig on my head. And, it looks pretty good.

Once again, kind and reassuring responses rolled in. I can't even count how many times I reread responses on Facebook to pick me up. My Facebook network became part of my daily inspiration.

> <u>Tammy</u> Keep finding the humor Holly.... the love and blessings and prayers are up to all of your friends and family- and there seems to be a PLETHORA of them!!!!!!!!!!!! xoxoxo

> <u>Carol B</u> Holly, I am so proud of you! You are my daily inspiration.
> My Aunt LaVenda was wearing a wig once when driving with a friend. Her friend had to jam on the brakes so suddenly that LaVenda's wig flew off into the back seat. We have laughed for years over that story. So, tip No.2 for your wig wearing....don't let anyone driving, stop the car suddenly!

> <u>Vicki</u> Hilarious! I'm glad you figured out how to put it on right. Although, maybe the punk rock look isn't so bad. Just toss on a Sex Pistols shirt and call it a day :)

> <u>Lorraine</u> It's gonna be all better in a few more months. No matter how much hair you have or how different you look in a wig -- it is absolutely still you. And we love you!!! There is no other person just like you in the universe.

> <u>Lorraine</u> P.S. If you have to eventually do eyebrows too, make sure you learn how to put them on right. That could really be freaky if they are crooked. : 0

> <u>Valerie</u> Go Holly! I'm w/ Vicki - I bet you

look hot as a punk rocker. Sorry to hear of your struggles, but so inspired by you for sharing them! We are all rooting for you!!

Shelley You got me! The first two paragraphs were sooo heavy and then I laughed out loud when I got the third. You'll get used to how you look, but it will take some time. It's hair...it will grow back! Stay strong my friend!

Dana Rachel told me that the purple wig was FABULOUS! You are amazing and look incredible with and without hair! Thanks for posting the note.

Ernie You look great PUNK! I would love to see pics with the purple wig, sounds fun.

Holly Toner-Rose Oh my gosh! You are all so wonderful! How lucky am I to have all of you? Thanks for the cheers. Hip Hip Hooray for Facebook friends!!!!

The responses went on and on like this. Again, all of these people lifting me up and carrying me though this dreadful experience was so appreciated. I can't thank you all enough for every last line of encouragement. It is those lines, and moments, and people that make you feel blessed to go through something like this.

That afternoon John picked up the girls from school. Not wanting to shock them I quickly went and put my wig on before they arrived back home. When they walked in and noticed my wig they both exclaimed that they loved it. Warning them first, I calmly explained that I had cut off my hair that day and then I pulled off my wig to show them. I wanted them to get used to the short hair before I was completely bald. I looked at each of them to gauge their responses. Hannah seemed okay. Her expression was not too extreme. Ivy's change in appearance was drastic. I watched her eyes bulge out of their sockets. I quickly put the wig back on and her eyes popped back into her head. This was going to take some time for us to get used to – for all of us.

For the rest of the evening the girls and I played board games. The girls still hadn't voiced their emotions at all about what was going on. I sensed they must have had glooming thoughts rolling about inside of them. How could they not? Their mother had breast cancer and was going through chemo. They had never seen me defeated like I had been the past few months, especially the past two weeks after my first round of chemo. Not only were they feeling the effects they were now seeing the effects. Now, Mommy no longer looked the same.

Trying to coax the girls to talk about it, I shared with them how I felt. I told them I thought it sucked that I didn't have hair anymore and it sucked that I got breast cancer. ("It sucks" is not a phrase we use often in our house, but I thought it was appropriate in this case and would help to make the point I wanted.) I told them that I thought they must have been feeling the same way. "Let's all shout it out. This sucks!" "Shout it out Ivy. Shout it out Hannah. It's okay honey. It's sucks!"

Ivy smiled as she shouted out loudly, "It SUCKS!"

Hannah more calmly in a monotone stated, "It sucks." She then asked me, "Why can't Mrs. Cadby's world be purple?"

I wanted to cry right then and there. My poor little girl. She didn't want Mrs. Cadby to be sick, but she didn't understand why it had to be her mommy that this was happening to. Why it had to be her that this was happening to. As I had been crying, "Why me? Why me?" my little girl had been crying the same tears. I loved her so much. I was going to get through this. She was going to get through. We all were.

We kept playing our board game. I called out "Hannah it's your turn." when I noticed fear in Ivy's eyes. "Ivy what's wrong baby?"

"What happened Mommy? What happened to your skin?" she said as she was pointing to my chest. She had just noticed my port for the very first time. She saw the three prongs from the plastic trying to poke their way out of my skin. I explained to her what it was and that it didn't hurt me. For the rest of the game she couldn't bear to look at me. She was horrified. I wanted to make it all better for Ivy and for Hannah, my sweet little girls.

I thought it might be helpful for Ivy to see everyone's Facebook responses to my new hairdo. The postings had had an amazing effect on my outlook and I thought they might do the same for her. I thought that if she realized other people actually liked my hair, she might like it too. I put her on my lap as I logged into Facebook. As it was loading, I explained that I wanted her to see something. When my profile picture popped up on the computer she gasped, "Mommy, don't put that picture on there!" She was mortified. There for all the world to see was her mommy looking like a monster.

I tried to reassure her, "Ivy, it's okay. People like it. Look at what people wrote about mommy's new haircut." I read a few of the better responses.

> Vicki You look stunning. If I shaved my hair down to the half-inch, people would run away from me screaming, 'fat marshmallow lady is coming to eat usssssssssssss.'

> Dan Holy shnikeys, you look great! Some serious PYT(pretty young thing). Let's get together for dinner this weekend. Soldier On Sister.

> Lorraine You do too look like you!! Shane said Aunt Holly can pull off any look!!

You look great!! I love you.

<u>Julie</u> Who needs hair when you have eyes that blue, cheekbones that really do look like apples and a smile like Holly Rose. You are so beautiful! All that hair was just hiding that pretty face. Your little light is shinin'

<u>Anita</u> OH My Holly! If we all could look as wonderful as you! You are so Beautiful, I love the cut Johnny gave you! You look great and you make me smile just looking at you!

It didn't change her mind. She wasn't buying it (neither was I). I hugged her and told her she could go play. That night I decided to keep my wigs on for Ivy. She needed to see mommy right now – not a monster - not cancer. I prayed for God to protect my little girls. To keep their minds safe. To keep me safe. I prayed.

Chapter Twenty-Four

Wednesday, April 15th, 2009. Wednesday was my normal day to have lunch with the girls at school and then help out. I didn't want to stop going to their school just because I had to wear a wig. This would be my first day at their school with a wig on. I wanted them to feel safe and secure so we made it fun.

The night before I told the girls any day I was going to their school they could pick out which wig I was going to wear. They both became excited about the prospect. Ivy quickly exclaimed, "The purple one! Wear the purple one."

Hannah jumped in with, "The Blonde one."

"No, the purple one." Back and forth they went. After a toss of a coin Ivy won and purple it was. Really it was a dark auburn, but in the sunlight it shone a hint of purple.

Nervously, I walked onto campus and went to check in. Unsure of myself I avoided all eye contact as I proceeded to Ivy's classroom. When I made my entrance all of the kids stared in amazement. Their eyes were wide open soaking up my new look and each of them wore a smile. One child quickly said, "I like your hair Mrs. Rose." And then another and another. Children are so beautiful. My confidence came back and so did Ivy's. She stood up next to me, proud to be by my side. Little did she know I was the one proud to be standing next to her.

Under the fresh sun we ate our lunch. The girls all excitedly asked me questions. "Why did I have to wear wigs? Did all of my hair fall out? Would it come back? How many wigs did I have? Would I wear my blonde one next week?" They went on and on. I was thrilled they asked every question. They asked every question Ivy wanted to ask but couldn't.

Smiling the girls left to go play on the playground. "Bye Mrs. Rose!" Before joining her friends Ivy gave me a big hug.

I hugged her back and told her, "I love you Ivy."

"I love you too, mom," she said as she skipped away. My baby was going to be okay.

Next was Hannah's group. Same thing. Wide eyes! Smiles! Compliments! She was going to be okay too. My sweet little girl.

I was now filled with positivity. The day before, I talked with Julie and we discussed how my experience was changing people's lives. I heard from my brother-in-law that my sister Sheree upon hearing the news that I had cancer had stopped complaining about her work. Her whole life was put into perspective. I told Julie how I had put my shaved head picture on Facebook and why. I wanted everyone to be grateful not just for their hair, but for their life. We talked about how wonderful it was that everyone in contact with me was appreciating life just a little bit more, even if only for a moment. I must admit that I felt a little proud of myself. I truly felt inspirational.

Later that afternoon I sat reading a book. The words I read made me realize how boastful I sounded and I was quickly humbled. Then, I recalled the adage Leslie had told me earlier that day, "It takes a village to raise a child." Her words rang true to me as well. I didn't deserve the credit for being an inspiration. It was my whole "village" that deserved the credit. My village and God. Not me. I felt arrogant and ashamed for ever having thought – "Yay, for me!" So many people had contributed to my voice. So many people were holding me up. I was just one piece of a beautiful puzzle that God had created.

A few days later our village congregated for the big day. It was Ivy's fourth grade field day.

Holly Toner-Rose loves Field Day Tug-O-War. PULL!! PULL!!

These were the days I loved. I looked forward to this just as much as Ivy did. I loved to see the kids running, laughing and skipping about. They all had victory in their eyes behind their youthful glow. Tweens at their best, every last one of them. I watched Ivy interacting with her friends. Her friends told me stories of this and that. I loved that they let me into their world.

It was a windy day and I was wearing my long blonde wig. The wig did not have hair in the center of it and was supposed to be worn with hats so that your head could breathe. I had my big floppy hat on with it that would have been great had it not been so windy. All day long I was fearful a strong gust of wind was going to blow my hat off and reveal my baldhead with an odd strap of hair around the circumference. Uncomfortable, I walked about chatting with other parents.

I started talking with one dad and I felt uneasy thinking he must be looking at my hair and wondering why I was wearing a wig. I awkwardly blurted out, "I just went through breast cancer treatment and chemo so I have to wear these wigs." Politely, he said he hadn't noticed (Why do I feel the need to do these things? I just embarrass the people I'm talking to and myself.)

The big event of the day was about to begin - the finale Tug-O-War. Class upon class struggling for the title. Ivy's class was last to go. Her teacher Mr. Sinclair, walked up and down the row repeating the strategy to the kids. "One, two, pull. . . One, two, pull…" I stood by Ivy trying to boost her and her friend's confidence with words of encouragement.

The flag was in place, the kids were eager and the bell rang out. Mr. Sinclair and I shouted out up and down the line, "ONE, TWO, PULL, ONE, TWO, PULL, ONE, TWO, PULL." The flag shimmied back and forth. Each child's grip was tight and the children's faces were contorted with determination. Some were leaning back with all their might and others who had lost control were still gripping tight but no longer part of the strength behind the momentum. "ONE, TWO, PULL, ONE, TWO, PULL."

I tried cheering them on but it looked as though they may be losing the battle. Inch by inch the flag started to move in the opposite direction towards the opposing team. And then I witnessed something incredible. Mr. Sinclair walked up and down the line screaming to the kids, "YOU ARE WINNING! YOU ARE TOTALLY WINNING! YOU ARE WINNING! ONE MORE PULL AND YOU ARE THERE." In one quick sentence he filled each and ever child with confidence and strength that was unbeatable. I watched the flag take leaps back toward their side. "YOU ARE WINNING," he shouted. And they won.

I took note that day what a little boost of confidence could do. How awesome would it be if I could do that every day with my children. I wanted to fill them with confidence that could carry them on for the rest of their lives. I was thankful that Ivy had Mr. Sinclair as a teacher. He built up the children every day. Ivy was lucky. We were lucky.

Hannah's field day was the following day. I was there to cheer her and her team on as well. I remembered Mr. Sinclair's strategy and I thought I'd put it to the test. As Hannah's class started to lose the battle I walked up and down screaming to each child, "YOU ARE WINNING! YOU ARE TOTALLY WINNING! YOU GOT IT! YOU'RE WINNING!" Low and behold her losing team gripped hard and pulled back again and again and won. They roared in victory. It was a beautiful sight to watch ten year olds jumping triumphantly. Life was good.

Later in that day I spoke with Gretchen. Her daughter Bridgette saw me out on the field cheering Ivy on the previous day. Bridgette didn't understand it. She asked, "Mom, how can Mrs. Rose be out there on the field during Tug-O-War when she is sick?" To a child there were no degrees of cancer. You were either healthy or sick. Having cancer meant you were sick. Cancer was scary. It was death. It was the big monster "C".

We had our fun at school with friends and now it was time for some family fun. We had planned to take the girls to Grandpa Marv's cabin for the weekend. As I was rushing around packing for the trip the strangest thing happened to me.

For weeks I had been worrying about what gave me cancer. "What did I need to change? What did I do wrong? What could have it been?" I never wanted to get this again. I didn't want to make the same mistake. Couldn't someone just tell me what it was that gave me cancer?????"

Standing at my vanity packing up my make-up I heard our front living room window shaking. The large window covered most of the twelve-foot room. A second time it shook even harder. For a brief second I thought that maybe we were having an earthquake, although we lived in Phoenix, Az., so that was unlikely. Fearful the window was going to break I ran to the room and then it suddenly stopped. I searched for an explanation, but I found nothing that could explain it.

Puzzled, I returned to my bedroom. The first thing I noticed when I went back to my vanity was the large jar of gold jewelry cleaner. I thought to myself "That's odd. I haven't used that in months. Why is it out?" Normally I kept it underneath my vanity cupboard tucked away in the back. Picking it up I read the label studying it. I couldn't pronounce many of the ingredients. Something prodded me to keep investigating.

I set the container down, opened up my vanity cupboard and was taken aback by the strong chemical smell. There behind my box of nail polishes was my container of silver cleaner. It had tipped over and it was lying on its side. My cupboard was saturated with the silver cleaner. I picked up the container, turned it towards the label and read, "This product contains chemicals known to cause cancer." I quickly dropped the jar of poison and ran to the bathroom, scrubbing my arms and hands.

"Oh my gosh! Is this what gave me cancer? I can't believe this. I've been breathing in cancer fumes every night for who knows how long. I can't believe I discovered this. I'm so lucky to have found this out. Wait a minute. My cleaner is never out. Why was it out? Why did the window shake? It was Janeen's ghost trying to tell me what gave me cancer. Oh my gosh!!!!!! Her ghost was trying to save me!!!!!!" (I have to laugh at myself now re-reading this.)

Quickly, I put on gloves, covered my face and cleaned up the toxic mess. Then I hurried and packed, excited for John to come home so I could tell him what happened. I wanted to call Janeen, Julie, Katie. . .someone to share my news that I just found out why I had cancer. Katie was the first to pick up. I recounted my "unbelievable story" to her. She is such a wonderful friend and said, "It's so good to know why you got cancer." (What she could have said is Holly you are a freak! No ghost came and told you the silver cleaner gave you cancer.)

Finally John came home with the girls and we packed up the car. We got in the car and I started to tell John my crazy story. . .The window shook. . .I never have my jewelry cleaner out. . . Hannah jumped in at this point, "Mom, I took that out today looking for nail polish remover."

"Wah. Wah. Wah." Her news somewhat killed my story. So maybe Janeen's ghost didn't try to tell me something or maybe she did. I don't know. I also don't know if fumes from the silver cleaner gave me cancer, or fumes from always painting gave me cancer, or smoking, or not eating healthy enough, or drinking too much alcohol, or cleaning chemicals, or the water or genetics or fate or what. I'll never know. All I know if that I don't want it again.

We arrived at the cabin ready to relax. It was the best nights sleep I had had in months. We enjoyed two days of rest and relaxation.

I asked John if on the way back home we could go through Sedona and go hiking and do a little shopping. Our friendly neighbor Chip lent us a book filled with Arizona hikes. He recommended a short hike in Sedona that ended with a view of Indian ruins.

The drive down through the switchbacks to Sedona was breathtaking. I marveled at the beauty God created around us. We arrived at lunchtime and we choose to eat at a grill with a spectacular view of the towering painted rocks surrounding us.

As we ate I talked about how excited I was to go on a hike. Hannah started to make fun of the idea of a hike and insinuated that she didn't want to go. I tried to convince her it was going to be fun. Stubbornly, she said she didn't want to hike. John followed suit jokingly. Ivy not wanting to be left out of the fun joined in. One by one they all commented on how lame the hike was going to be.

I was cursing them all in my mind, "How dare they? Do they have any idea what I just went through the past week? Do they have any idea? No they don't, because I did my best to try to hide the symptoms and not complain about it! I tried to protect everyone. And now I'm asking for one hike. Are they kidding me?"

And they continued to complain about going on a hike. "And John, he should know better. After all I've done for everyone and I'm going through cancer and chemo and they can't go on one hike with me!!!! Lazy pigs!!!! They would be happy to have their minds dissolve into the TV. Well not me. I want to live. Has John not learned anything from my experience with cancer? Does he not care about living? Or me?? I guess not. I'll go hike by myself!"

As they joked back and forth to one another I glared at them all, while trying to keep my tears back. "Fine, You don't have to go. But I'm going." As I said it, my efforts to hold back tears were futile.

In my mind I whimpered, "Just one. Just one. Damn it. I don't want to cry. Just one." John looked over at me with shame in his eyes. He turned foot and told the girls we were all going hiking and that was that.

We arrived at the trail and John led the way and the girls and I followed. "Look at me. I'm hiking. You can't get me cancer. I'm living," I thought to myself.

We walked on finding the steep trail leading up to the rainbow arch, where the book mentioned the ruins would be. John and Hannah started up the trail with Ivy and me lagging behind. Ivy had her musical elephant, Elliot, in tow.

Elliot was Ivy's stuffed elephant she received as a gift the day she was born. If you pulled his tail down he would play a song. She had that little elephant clasped tightly near her for the first two year of her life. We couldn't leave the house without him and if we did we immediately turned around to go retrieve him. He was Ivy's security blanket. And now after years of sitting on her shelf, Elliot was once again in tow everywhere Ivy went, including our hike in Sedona.

On the hike John repeatedly asked if I was okay. I told him I was fine and that I'd let him know if I had to go back. Slowly, I clambered up each giant rock. I could still feel the chemo pumping through my body. Panting it out of my lungs and through my esophagus I breathed out invisible clouds. My heart beat faster. Up and up I went. "I'm going to do this. Damn it. I'm going to do this. I can do this. I can." And finally we reached the top.

We all sat in the shade resting our tired bodies from our short hike. Hannah, not so worn out, jumped up and said, "Let's climb to the top to find the ruins." Wanting to see them too I jumped up to join her. I took three steps and realized I was not doing so well. I thought I was going to faint. Quickly, I sat back down.

I thought to myself, "Crap! What did I just do? Let's go on a hike? What was I thinking? I just did chemo a week ago? I shouldn't be hiking on some isolated trail? Crap. I have to make it back down. What if I faint going down? What was I thinking!!!!! That was SO not smart of me! Crap!!!! Okay, I'll be okay. I'll rest a bit and I'll be okay."

We sat there in the shade for ten minutes and then John decided it was time to head back. I didn't mention that I thought I was going to faint. I just marched on. There was no need to scare everyone, myself included. Every step my head was spinning. Microwave brain waves started to vibrate through my skull. My heart raced spitting out chemo residue. "Crap. What if I faint up here? No one can even get to me. John can't carry me down this steep rocky path. I have to make this." Step by step by step I told myself, "I can do this. I can do this. Just keep going Holly. You are going to be okay. You can do this." And I did. By the time I made it to the clearing I was completely exhausted. Now I just had a short flat path to the car.

Once we reached the path I told John I wasn't doing good. "I feel like I'm going to faint honey."

"I KNEW we shouldn't have done this," he said. I agreed with him this time. I held onto his shoulder for support and we slowly walked along. Every few minutes I had to sit and rest. In my mind I started thinking how embarrassing it would be if a rescue team had to come take me out. My pace became slower and slower. John noticed and stopped. He told me to get on his back and I didn't resist one little bit. He lowered himself and I jumped on and he piggybacked me out of there. He was my hero once again.

We drove home feeling the Vortex of Sedona. Life was good. Our family was good.

Chapter Twenty-Five

Prior to my third round of chemotherapy Alisha brought me soup and more sitcoms to pass the time along with a nutrition book she thought I might like. Alisha had been so helpful and caring. She came every week with more soup or cleaning supplies ready to clean and ears to listen. Her and Brenda both.

I spent the next few days reading the nutrition book. I decided I was going to take every precaution I could to ensure that this would never come back. If it did come back it wouldn't be because of anything I had done or not done. After everything I read I concluded I needed to give up a few things. I decided to quit eating red meat, quit drinking diet coke, become vigilant in my five fruits and veggies a day, organic of course, cut out processed foods, drink fifty percent of my body weight in water a day, exercise, and anything else I read that could possibly help. I had my work cut out for me.

> Holly Toner-Rose has given up red meat
> but will never give up my coffee.

That night I had yet another dream. In this one five ninja's dressed in black kept chasing me trying to kill me. One man in black, named John, appeared every time, fighting off the villainous mob and saving me. I went to the man and paid him five hundred dollars for his help in protecting me. I asked him, "Will they stop? Will they ever stop? You can't always be there for me when they appear out of nowhere."

He replied, "They will never stop. Never. The only thing you can do is move off the beach."

"That is five blocks." (In my dream we were living back in San Diego on the beach.) I immediately went to find John to let him know it was imperative that we moved and quickly. I found the girls at home alone and grabbed them both.

I left a note for John and headed out. We had to get going before the pack of ninja's hunting me down returned. Unfortunately, I can't remember the ending of the dream.

So for my interpretation of what I do remember: Chemo was trying to kill my body. I had endless packs of chemo cells inside of me all wanting to kill me. John kept me alive each round, nurturing my body and spirit. I was indebted to him, but would he be able to do that forever if I had to go through chemo again? I needed a new approach.

I thought about the repetition of the fives. What was that all about? I came up with there must be five things I must change. Five things I needed to be doing differently in my life. What else? What else did I need to change? What was number five? What was number five? I had changed my diet drastically. I cleaned up the jewelry cleaner and abolished any other cleaners in my house that were not organic. I also rid our home of any products in our house that were not organic. I threw out hundreds of dollars of lotions, shampoos, deodorants, etc. I had also rearranged our house to Feng Shui standards.

At some point I came home with a Feng Shui book and one of the first pages I turned to informed me that the exact way my bed was positioned and being placed underneath the window and with direct access to view another bedroom door the person occupying the space in the bed on the left was sure to contract a serious disease. That was my space. After reading this I immediately went to rearranging our bedroom. And reading more I had to rearrange more - pictures, and colors and mirrors . . . Everything was off! What was I to do? Maybe I did need to move! John quickly stole the book away from me to cease my nervous and needless rearranging and worry.

For the next few days I focused what energy I had on Hannah and Ivy and John. I was no longer the doting wife and mother I used to be. My energy was spent fighting the effects of chemo. Everyone was sacrificing on my behalf. I watched the girls slowly distancing themselves from me. I'm sure it was their natural instincts kicking in to protect themselves, but it sure did hurt. I was hurting inside and out.

Ivy was still having a hard time with me being bald. She interpreted everything visually and now I didn't look like mommy. I watched her pull away from me day after day. I was a stranger, a scary ugly stranger. I tried to always wear a wig in Ivy's presence. If I had a wig on she would still come to me, hug me, cuddle me . . . If I wasn't wearing a wig she kept her distance. I could feel her pulling away as I would hug her and she kept her eyes averted. It broke my heart. I understood, but it still broke my heart.

John at one point told her, "You need to tell Mommy she doesn't have to wear the wigs or the scarves. They are uncomfortable for Mommy." She came to me and repeated his words. I knew though that in her heart she didn't want to see me without a wig. I scared her. Mommy scared her. John wanted me to be comfortable and protect me, but I didn't care about myself. I cared about my baby and she needed to see me with hair.

Hannah seemed to by okay with me losing my hair. She didn't mind looking at my bald head or touching it. I was still Mommy, hair or no hair. In fact, Hannah found a way to have fun with it. She took my brush that was overflowing with hair from the day my hair started to fall out. She decided she wanted to make a craft out of my hair. She constructed a diorama in a box depicting a school cafeteria that included a lunch line with a crabby cafeteria worker, donning my hair of course and a scared child, again with my hair.

She proudly marched into her classroom with her completed diorama and requested to display it. The school was so accommodating to my baby that they displayed her masterpiece right there in the cafeteria for all to see. Proudly, I took pictures of her creation and posted them on Facebook, "Hannah's fun with human hair!" She too was finding something good in the horrific. She painted my world purple once more.

Round three was nearing so we tried to capture a little more of life. We made plans to go out to dinner with Katie and her friend Shane. John and I arrived early to watch the sunset on the rooftop. It was so nice to be alone with him relaxing. Something we hadn't done much of lately. It almost felt like nothing was wrong for a second.

We both enjoyed a glass a red wine and each other's company. The wine soothed our tense bodies, relaxing every muscle as it swam through our veins. We had both been under so much stress. We needed this.

Katie and Shane arrived and we decided to have another glass of wine with them. We were feeling so good, why not? We deserved a little enjoyment. By the time we finished the second glass we were all laughing having a great time. It felt so refreshing to be doing something normal - out to dinner with friends. I wanted everything to be normal again. I didn't want to go back for more tomorrow. I wasn't ready. I wanted to live - damn it. I had just started to feel normal and now I have to go back tomorrow and feel like utter crap for another week.

We sat and contemplated another glass of wine. If we had another we would have to taxi home. I told John, "I'm going to feel like crap anyway tomorrow. What the hell? Let's have fun!" And we did. We ordered another glass and then another. We all stumbled into the taxi and topped if off with one more glass at Katie's house. We arrived home and I clumsily fell out of the taxi and onto my face. It was not a pretty sight. John and I had tried to squeeze in two months worth of fun into one night.

Thursday, April 23rd, 2009. I awoke the next morning with the worst red wine hangover of my life. Looking in the mirror I discovered a dark bruise and skid mark on my cheek from falling out of the taxicab. "What was I thinking? How stupid can I be? I have to go do chemo now? What if all the alcohol in my system screws it all up and something goes wrong? Crap! I have to tell them! Who gets drunk the night

281

before chemo? What the hell is wrong with me? Aaaaahhhhhh! I'm such an idiot!"

Walking into chemo I held my head down in shame. Nervously, I thought, "What the hell do I say? I have to say something. I can't NOT say something. A nurse walked by me, glanced at my eye and asked what happened. I told her I tripped and fell in my new purple high heel shoes (I did trip and fall, I just left out the part that I fell out of a taxi cab drunk).

Brie, my chemo nurse, walked over and starting flushing out my port. I told her, "I'm afraid I did something awful last night that I have to tell you."

Her eyes widened with anticipation. "What?" I proceeded to tell her my story of one glass, then two, then my theory of what the hell I'm going to feel like crap anyway so let's have fun. "Oh, that's all. I thought you were going to tell me something really bad. The wine will just thin out your blood a little, that's all, and give you a bad headache." I was so relived. I vowed never to do that again.

I sat through another round of chemo with a hangover. I felt awful the whole time, but then again I did every time I had chemo. I was right after all. It didn't really matter.

As I sat there in my lazy-boy I thought to myself that is number five. That was the fifth thing I needed to change - alcohol. Alcohol had not been a big part of my life since college . . . since I met John. I could take it or leave it. Alcohol had somehow snuck back into my life in the past year or two.

I never had a problem with an occasional wild night out on the town, but lately it was becoming more and more frequent. There always seemed to be an occasion for alcohol; a dinner party, a meeting at the county club, a birthday celebration, girl's night out. Everything we went to socially involved alcohol. One glass of wine became two and two became three and then some. I was on the road to becoming an alcoholic. I thought to myself that maybe this was all a blessing in disguise. I was a little relived we now had an out of the heavy drinking activity. (I was given another blessing in disguise when I read in my oncologist office that women who have had breast cancer increased their risk of reoccurrence by thirty percent if they consume more than three glasses of alcohol a week. And women with no history of breast cancer and drink more than seven glasses of alcohol in a week increase their risk by thirty percent.) So my wild drinking days were long gone. Again, I think this was a blessing in disguise. John quit drinking as well. Our life together is much better with the absence of alcohol.)

Time passed slowly as I contemplated my regrets and finally another was round completed.

With each passing treatment my mental state weakened. I tried to stay positive but it was getting more and more difficult. The couch became my permanent spot during my chemo coma as I watched life move by me. I watched the girls living and I watched John living. I was not living. Chemo had killed my spirit. Worst of all it killed my parenting skills. I was no longer a good mother.

Late Sunday afternoon while lying on the couch I watched Hannah bound in from the other room smiling ear to ear. She had finally finished the play she was writing for school. She stood in front of me with her proud smile and papers in hand ready to show off her hard work. Before she could even begin I asked her if she had finished her other homework and I started to scold her for not finishing it. I watched the smile on her face dissolve and a frown appear. I instantly realized how disheartening I made my daughter feel. I caused that. No one else. Me! The one who was supposed to build her up just tore her down.

I tried to backup for a redo. With Hannah sitting next to me I cried out, "I'm so sorry Hannah. That was soooo wrong of Mommy! I really want to hear your play. I'm so proud you. Will you please read it to me?"

Her eyes averted away from me as she said, "I don't want to now."

I held her paper in my hands pleading with her, "Please Hannah! I'm so sorry honey."

With disappointment in her voice she flatly stated, "No, I don't want to."

As tears rolled down my cheeks spotting her paper with watermarks I pleaded again, "Please Read It! PLEASE."

Desperately wanting to go back in time I cried out to her. "I'M SORRY HANNAH! I'M SO SORRY! WILL YOU PLEASE READ IT!!!!! PLEASE!!!"

At that point I was sobbing and hysterically crying out how bad of a mother I was and incapable of nurturing my children, "I hate this. I hate chemo. I hate cancer. I can't be a good mom anymore. I can't! I can't! I'm so sorry! I'm losing it! I'M LOSING IT! I CAN'T DO THIS!" John walked over with a loving look in his eye and picked me up off the couch and carried me into our bedroom.

"Oh my biliken. Your faced is all screwed up when you cry. No more tears." He then carried me into the bathroom and he sat me down on the floor and turned on the faucet to the bath. He turned to me and said, "It's okay Holly. It's gonna be okay Holly.

He left me alone to soak away my tears. I sat with my big bald head, clutching my knees watching the water spew out, knowing it wasn't going to wash anything away. I was now a bad mother. The thing I loved most of all. It was all so unfair. I worked so hard to be a good person, to be a good wife, to be a good mom and now I wasn't good at any of it. None of it. All of it taken away from me in one swoop. All of it! I didn't want this anymore. I couldn't do this anymore. I wanted it all to be over. There was nothing I could do but wait for another day to pass, and another and another.

I lay back in the tub hoping to find escape. I didn't. I listened to the strong pounding of my heart desperately trying to push the killer chemo out of my body. It pumped harder and harder and louder and louder. It did nothing to soothe my fragile nerves. John was the only person who soothed me. He made it all better for me. He always did. Whenever I needed him he was there.

John tucked me in bed and kissed away my tears. He reassured me it was going to be okay. Hannah did indeed read me her play and it was magnificent. She was magnificent and she forgave me and my faux pas and the many more that followed. They all did. I love them so.

Chapter Twenty-Six

<u>Holly Toner-Rose</u> is ready for round 4. I'm halfway there.

<u>Tammy</u> Thinking of you and cheering you on Holly.

<u>Valerie</u> Yes, hang in there! Sending you lots of love.

<u>Jeremy</u> So very proud of you honey! Your a real trooper and def. someone i admire!!!!!~michelle

<u>Jennifer</u> Half way already. Awesome!

Wednesday May 6th, 2009, the day prior to my next round of chemo. Ivy excitedly told me about her band concert that was the following evening. She was playing the stand up bass. I thought about the many instruments blaring, while my head would be tightening, my wigs would become more and more uncomfortable like a tight wool sweater that was two sizes too small worn in the heat of summer, and the zaps of microwave brain shocking my brain. I wasn't sure I would be able to sit through it.

With Ivy sitting across from me I regretfully said, "Ivy, I don't know if Mommy can make it tomorrow. I have my chemo day tomorrow." Ivy knew full well what chemo day meant. It was the beginning of one week of hell for me and her and the rest of our family. It was one week of uncertainty. One week of confusion and disorder. One week of misery.

Ivy looked up at me with disappointment in her eyes and said, "It's okay Mommy. You don't have to go." The heavy look of sadness in her flowery eyes hurt me more than the chemo did. I couldn't let my baby down. Microwave brain or not I was going to be there to watch my baby perform.

Promising her I would be there the next day, I held her close to me and told her how much I loved her. She smiled. I did make it to Ivy's concert and she played beautifully. My eyes filled with pride and love for my baby, even though my head was filled with toxins and pain.

I survived the next five days and conquered yet another round. On Tuesday I sat with my feet in the pool watching the girls swim all day. I could feel strep throat coming on again. Chemo was breaking down my body. This was the second time strep throat attacked me during chemo.

I wasn't too concerned in the morning. I did what I was supposed to do - I called the chemo nurse and waited for them to return my call informing me they had called in medicine to my pharmacy. Hours went by and still no call.

At 4:00 desperate for some relief I called back and all they did was make me an appointment with a P.A. for the next day.

That night was the worst experience. I tossed and turned in agonizing pain. The swelling of my tonsils caused intense pain to my ears, especially my right ear and there was nothing I could do about it. First, I tried every sleeping position I could think of - no relief. I tried medicines - no relief. I broke out the heating pad and slept with it pressed up firmly against my ear – no relief. I sobbed, "It hurts. It hurts John. I'm in so much pain. It feels like my ear is going to explode. I just want to sleep." I whimpered my way through the night crying.

Finally, my night of agony ended. John drove me to the doctor's office. "Those damn doctors! Why didn't they give you something!" He grabbed my hand and told me it would be better soon. Finally, we made it to the office and like a sick little puppy I slowly made my way to the door.

We walked down the long hallway only to find the door locked. There was a note on the door that stated they were having electrical problems. I didn't care about electrical problems I just needed a prescription to make my pain go away. I sat down in front of the door, holding my ear trying to ease the pain, while John pounded on the door. Someone finally made their way to the door and asked John for my info to reschedule me for another day. "Were they out of the minds? My ear was going to explode any second. I was in pain here. I couldn't wait another day or take another night of what I had been through before." She told us we could go across the street to the hospital. This didn't seem like much of an option since hospitals usually had a four to six hour waiting game of its own. John drove away, me in tears and him in a swearing fit. In between his swearing he called doctors trying to get me an appointment.

John called our primary care physician who was understaffed that day and was not able to get us in. He drove me to the Urgent care office. I slowly walked in, signed in and took my seat for the two-hour plus wait. John was still outside on the phone, cussing up a storm to someone. I laid my head back against the wall not caring if it tilted my wig one bit. I was in too much pain to care about my wig or anyone around me. Then I realized it was time to play the chemo card.

Since my treatment began I had not used the chemo card once. I never wanted to receive special treatment or have people feel sorry for me because I was going through chemo, but this time I was going to use it. In my head I was working up my courage to storm to the front desk, pull off my wig and explain loudly, "I'm in pain here and not just my ear either. There is no way I can tolerate sitting her for two hours waiting when the acid diarrhea will be hitting me soon and my microwave head hasn't stopped for five days, and my bones feel like they are rotting from the inside out and the nasal drip is next and I have to go back in for another round in eight days. I NEED TO SEE A DOCTOR NOW"

And then my hero, John, walked in and said, "Let's go honey. I got them to call you in some medicine." John came through for me once again. I never would have been able to do that.

John had always been able to convince people to do things. He has something about him that makes people want to please him. People like him and want his affection and attention. It's a gift really. This is a gift I do not possess and I love about him.

I've always felt so honored that he chose me. There were many a girl who chased him, but he never noticed the other women because he only had eyes for me. I had to overcome my jealousy early on when girl after girl would bat their eyes at him in front of me. And believe me this was not an easy task for me with all of my insecurities topped off with blonde tan bikini babes walking the streets of San Diego. They were at every turn. They swooned around him with me near by turning green. Talking myself out of a jealous rage each time with the help of a few prayers I would tell myself, "If he wants someone else there is nothing I can do about it. If he wants me he will choose me. And Lucky me he did!

I realized that one of the beautiful things I discovered during cancer was a renewed sense of love and admiration for John. He had been my hero from the day that I met him on the beach of Mexico. I still believe we had guardian angels bring us together. It was fate. He was my hero. Somewhere along the way, between diapers and naps and moving and struggling, I forgot this. While going through cancer it slapped me in the face again. He was still my hero. He always had been. Nothing had changed. He hadn't changed. I hadn't changed. Life just put on a few blinders for a while. I was ashamed that I let life do this to me. John is a great man, a great husband and great father. How lucky was I? I could be wrong, but I don't think most people are given this gift in life - To really see who it was they fell in love with and why eighteen years later. I was lucky and in love.

Holly Toner-Rose is lucky, lucky, lucky me!

The weekend came and it was time for another cousin sleepover. John and I loved having the cousins over to play. The time was wholesome and pure and filled our family with warm fuzzies.

In the middle of the night I heard "Bluuuh! Bluuuuh! Bluuuuh!" Someone was throwing up. Instinctively, I ran to the other side of the house and stopped myself at the bathroom door. I new my immune system was compromised and I was afraid of contracting anything new.

Hannah was throwing up. I called out to her "Oh baby! I'm so sorry! Mommy, can't be near you. I can't get sick honey." "JOHN! JOHN!" John was there in an instant. He mopped up the barf on the floor, the toilet and on Hannah. I stood in the hallway sending my soothing sympathies her way. My mind was filled with grief. Here was my baby throwing up and I couldn't even stand next to her and hold up her hair, and calm and soothe her little aching body. I couldn't be the mommy that I had been in the past. Even if I tried I just couldn't. It broke my heart.

I was proud of John as I watched him jump in and play my part without hesitation and he played it well. The girls depended on him now, not me. I was replaceable. I just wanted this to all be over and done with. I wanted to be a good Mommy again. My heart hurt watching my role dissolve in their eyes. My body hurt, my mind hurt . . . my heart hurt.

Monday May 18th, 2009. John's mom, Carol, was in town. Her and Brenda came over to clean our house. I couldn't have been more appreciative. Again, I couldn't do it myself. Physically, I just couldn't. John and the girls had enough on their plates keeping up with life along with all of their added duties, the stress of all the recent changes and new fears was all they could handle. Carol and Brenda were my angels for the day folding ever last load and scrubbing every last tile. I needed their help. I needed everyone's help.

Carol and Brenda asked during lunch how I was doing? I was tired of telling everyone I was okay and it wasn't so bad.

I wasn't okay. It was bad. It was not just bad it was HORRIBLE! So, I told them the truth. I told them every God awful detail of what chemo was doing to my body. Their faces froze upon hearing my shocking details, even Carol's. Maybe I should have just stuck to I was okay and it wasn't so bad.

We changed the subject and Brenda shared some of the things that her husband did that drove her crazy. I shared too. I told them that one time when John was mad at me he went around the house and move things just enough to off center them. He moved pictures, vases, etc. It didn't take me long to notice that things were out of place. It drove me crazy!!!!!!

I told them "That's okay, cuz when I get mad at John, I dry his shirts." John likes to hang dry his t-shirts. (They are t-shirts, just dry the darn things.)

"And when I'm really mad, I pinch him in his sleep." Brenda about fell off her chair when I told her this one.

"What do you mean you pinch him? Does he wake up?"

"Well yeah, cuz I pinch him really hard on his chest. Then I feel better and by the time he wakes up he's forgotten about it." We all laughed and laughed. I laughed my misery away. My house was clean, my mind was clean. Life was good.

Later that day I planned for the girls to have their end of the year swim party at our house. We did this every year to celebrate the end of the school year and the coming of summer. I wasn't going to have this year be any different for them. We had a house full of happy tweens swimming and playing and dancing and screaming for two hours straight. My eyes were still seeping with chemo drip and I was exhausted, but I didn't care one bit, my girls were having fun. The fun finally came to an end and everyone went home.

As we sat at the dinner table I asked if the girls had a good time. Each of them nonchalantly said, "Yah."

That was it. "Yah."

"Were they kidding? Did they have any idea what it

took for me to put together a party in the shape that I was in. And now, not one Thank You! Not One!" I was angry and hurt and disappointed all at the same time.

After dinner I told John how I was feeling and he discouraged me from scolding them. "They are tired too Holly. They appreciate it. They just forgot to say it this once."

He was right, but it did hurt my feelings. I had pushed myself for them and didn't receive an ounce of recognition for it. Maybe that was just me being selfish though. I didn't plan the party for recognition. I planned it so they could have fun and they did. Why was I mad then? Why did I want recognition so badly then? Maybe it was because I had felt like I had become a bad mother during chemo. I wanted them to reinstate me to my "good mom" status and they didn't.

Chapter Twenty-Seven

Thursday May 21st, 2009. Today was chemo number five. It was time for my second drug of treatment. I was receiving Taxol for the next four rounds. I heard from all of the chemo nurses that Taxol was much easier than the Adriamiacin I had received for my first four rounds. I was hoping and praying this was true.

As I sat in my easy chair waiting for the nurse to get me going I overhead the woman next to me talking with the nurse. She must have been close to eighty. She reminded me of the older woman in Pollyanna who always complained. In her nasally, negative voice she said, "I'm not going to make it to Christmas. There's no way I'm going to make it to then." Her son interrupted her and said he'd return when she was done with chemo. I glanced over at her and all I could see was her years. Years of living life, years with her children, with her husband . . . years. That was all I wanted. I had prayed and bargained and begged God for years. I was hoping and praying I would make it to sixty-five. If I could just make it to sixty-five my girls would be okay without me and so would John. It would be okay.

I wanted to tell her, "Do you know how lucky you are? How fortunate you are you to have lived as long as you have? I'd give anything, ANYTHING, in this world to have the guarantee that I will live to be sixty-five." I wanted to tell her to be grateful and stop complaining – but I didn't. I smiled and opened up my laptop ready for another round of sitcoms to take my mind away from her and everything else.

Hours later I returned home and waited. Waited for symptoms. Would they come? What would they be this time around? Would they be worse? How long would they last? I waited.

I felt a little nauseous but nothing too bad. I had refused early on to take some of the anti-nausea medicine. Most of them were steroids that I didn't care to put in my body and one of their side effects was weight gain. That was all I needed. Let's feel crappy during chemo and now let's feel crappy about how I look too. Like being bald wasn't enough they wanted to give me meds to make me fat too. No thanks. I can deal with a little nausea.

The next morning I woke up craving my cup of coffee. Any time I can drink coffee I know I'm not that sick. Four rounds of this – piece of cake. I made my morning post of Facebook.

> Holly Toner-Rose has woken up before her whole family and is enjoying the morning silence with a big cup of java. Aaahhhh! Now this is the life.

And then the pain set it. It came on like a ton of bricks. One minute I was cleaning going about the day with a smile on my face and the next minute I realized my bones were starting to ache, and the next I felt a flood of exhaustion come over me, and the next I was down. Down for days.

My bones felt like someone was hollowing them from the inside out, scraping out any cancer inside. Each and every last bone from my toes, to my legs, to my back to my arms to my knuckles, every single one ached. I would make my way to a super hot bath trying to soak the pain away. The bath would work for a few instants and then the pain would start to return. I tried this at least three times a day.

And the exhaustion was overwhelming. I had never experienced anything like it. Making my way out of the bathtub to my bed was like marching across the Sahara desert. I would collapse by the time I reached my bed. Keep in mind that the distance from my bathtub to my bed is maybe twenty-five feet. Before I could dress myself I would have to rest for a few minutes to regain strength. From there I would have to rest again before making my way back to the couch.

A few of the other symptoms that went along with

Taxol were swelling of my tonsils, but I found a great remedy for that one. Grape juice slushies like the ones I made in the summertime as a child. I just had to pour grape juice in a plastic cup, place it in the freezer for four to five hours, and viola! you had a slushy. I slurped these down by the hour. They were the one and only thing that soothed my throat.

Nasal drip poured out of my eyes for days. This didn't come on until day five and when it did it looked like I always had tears in my eyes for a week. I also had chemo burps. My husband loved this one. Out of nowhere and with no warning my body let out a tiny little chemo burp. It tasted like chemo and smelled like chemo. It was making its final round through my body and out my mouth. This was taxol for me. Four rounds.

Thursday, May 28th 2009. This was the girls' first day of summer. My spirits picked up a bit with summer. My babies were home to make me laugh and smile. They took care of me. Hannah would periodically sit next to me and rub my big baldhead. She even drew a picture of me with my baldhead and she gave me a halo and the caption read, "Holly Rose is the best mom in the world, even without her long hair." Ivy had even gotten over her fear of my baldhead. She still didn't want to hug me if I didn't have my wig on but she wasn't afraid anymore. I was with Ivy. I still hated it.

I would catch a glimpse of myself on occasion walking past a mirror and I saw a creepy crawly creature right out of a fantasy novel. I was a creature - No wonder Ivy didn't want to hug me. I quit caring what I looked like at home though. I just didn't look at myself. I had to go with comfort even if I did look monstrous. I had too many other ailments to have to worry about my head being hot because of a wig on top of it.

I continued on as best as could. We all did. I made my posts on Facebook and counted down the days.

Holly Toner-Rose knows this sounds silly, but I'm so excited I just mopped my floor. It's the first time in 3 months. No, I'm not that lazy, and yes other people have mopped my floor. It's just the first time I've felt physically up for it. Yay!!!!! (Never thought I'd say that.)

Holly Toner-Rose has rediscovered her favorite childhood sick remedy. Grape juice slushies!

Holly Toner-Rose loves summer!!!!!!

Holly Toner-Rose is thankful.

Holly Toner-Rose 35 days and counting!!!!

Holly Toner-Rose I need some serious exercise. All of my muscle is turning to flab. It's not pretty.

Holly Toner-Rose is thinking I've wasted my whole morning on Facebook. It's time to go out and live.

Holly Toner-Rose is going into round 7 with only one more round to go after this. I think I can! I think I can! I think I can! I see the top of the mountain!!!!!!

It was the day before my next chemo. I wanted to go out a live. I needed exercise to fight the demons in my head, so I decided to go for a walk down the bridle path with the girls. We all jumped in the car and picked up cousin Maddy on the way. Maddy proceeded to tell us about the little dog that they were trying to find a home for. I had always been adamant that we were not getting a dog. I had two kids to care for and that was all I could handle. Another puppy was like having another child. A dog was the last thing I needed. Here I was in the middle of chemo though, condemned to my couch for a week at a time, while the rest of my family was living life. Maybe I did need a puppy.

On our walk the girls pleaded and pleaded, "We'll take

care of it. We'll feed it and walk it and pick up the poop."

I finally broke down and said, "We can take him home and try him out for one day. How about that?"

"Yay!!!!!"

Finished with our short walk we went to drop off Maddy and pick up our tester puppy. As I stepped out of the car, cousin Andy came walking outside their front door with a big ball of fluff. I ran over picked up the puppy exclaiming, "Oh, this is Sooooo our puppy." And that was that. We were now a dog family. The proud owners of a little Pomeranian. He was our little fluff-ball of love. Now he just needed a name. We took a family vote and unanimously picked John's entry Bobo. Bobo was our new little baby.

Cuddling with our new baby we all watched a TV show that described different phobias. One of the many phobias they covered was the fear of the number thirteen. People that suffered from this had triskaidekaphobia. I was included in this class. I almost cancelled a flight when they told me my seat was number 213. "Were they kidding? Who puts the number thirteen anywhere on a plane or anywhere else for that matter?" I had receptionists trying to make me appointments in the past year on the thirteenth. "Again, were they kidding? Yeah, I want my first visit with my chemo doctor on the thirteenth. Are they crazy??????" Looking back over my experience I realized after reviewing my writing that the original posting I viewed reminding me to perform a self-breast exam was on January 13th and I lost my hair on April 13th, my nightmare strep throat with the Dr.'s office closed was on the thirteenth . . . I most definitely feared the number thirteen.

HollyToner-Rose has triskaidekaphobia.

Chapter Twenty-Eight

Thursday, July 2nd 2009. It was a day to celebrate. I stood in front of the mirror applying my make-up when I noticed a teeny tiny hair above my upper-lip. A HAIR! I took a closer look and discovered another and then another. Hair was growing back on my body. I reached for the top of my head rubbing ever so lightly and I felt the sparse beginnings of fuzz. "HAIR! YAY! HAIR! I'm going to have hair again. Thank you God!"

Holly Toner-Rose doesn't mind one bit that my mustache hair is coming back because my hair is coming back. HAIR!!! HAIR!!! GLORIOUS HAIR!!!!!!!!!

Jennifer , Nicole and 2 others like this.

Alissa Still red and curly? You GROW, girl! Hurrah!

Jasmine Whoo hoo!!!!!!

Marina Nice!

Hillary You're such a superSTAR!!

Kim yah hair!

I was also celebrating that fact that today was my last round of chemo. We sent our girls off to the cabin with all of their cousins and Aunts and Uncles. There was no need for them to go through one last round. They had already been through enough.

As I sat in my lazy chair for my final four hours of treatment I prayed this would be the last time I would be there. I prayed it would be my last round of chemo forever. I wanted to live again. I wanted to be a good mom and wife again. I wanted to feel like me again. I said goodbye to all of the nurses and went home and waited.

I waited for the final round to kick in thinking it might be easier this time knowing it was the last, but it wasn't. It was just as hard as every other round. Five days filled with intense bone pain and utter exhaustion. John remained by my side every day reminding me, "This is the last round Holly. You did it. You only have a couple days to go and it's all over. We're leaving on vacation in a couple of days." A couple more days and I could live again.

> Holly Toner-Rose YAY!! YAY!!! I DID IT!!! 4 MONTHS OF CHEMO-I'M DONE!!! YAY!! YAY!!! YAY!!! YAY!!! I DID IT!!!!!!!!!!!!!! Thank you everyone for all of your support through this. I couldn't have made it through without you all!! THANK YOU!!!!!!

I had my whole network with me all the way to the finish line cheering me on!

> Dan , Jennifer , Marina and 2 others like this.

> Jeremy I'm soooooooooooo proud of you holly-congrats again!!!!!!!!!!~Michelle

> Anna Holly Toner Rose you are an amazing woman!!!

> Kim Proud of you girl! Congrats for kicking butt through all of this!

> Joe CONGRATS!

> Kristine I am thrilled for you! Now go, have an excellent vacation!!

> Tonya You're awesome and inspiring!

> ArinHooray for you Holly!!! I can't wait until I can say the same thing! Thanks for the inspiration!

Valerie Great news, Holly! You are such an inspiration. Can't wait to see you in a couple weeks!!!

Alisha Yes!!!!!!!!

Shelley Holly...you managed to survive such a difficult situation with such grace and humor. I am very proud of you and you are a role model to us all!

Jeanne So happy to hear that! Hope to see you guys soon! :)

Kimmie I'm so glad to hear that! I'm sure it wasn't easy but you seemed to make the best out of it and that's what makes you a great person and mom

Anita Congratulations! I am so proud of you Holly! Have a wonderful celebration and holiday!

Sheree Yipee you're finally done...love ya

Jennifer Woo Hoo!!!!!!!!!!!!!!!!!

Hillary you are such an inspiration!!

Jenn great job holly! now go have some fun!

Christopher YOU are strong one!

Jerry Congratulations! I'm so happy for you.

I'm not sure how I would have gotten through my four months of chemo without everyone's support. Someone was always there picking me up and cheering me on. I was overflowing with gratitude for everyone!

Friday, July 10th 2009. We left for our two-week vacation. We all desperately needed this. Our stress levels had all been so high for so long. We needed to relax, to laugh . . . to enjoy life. I had endured four months of chemo and it was over. It was all over. I was ready to celebrate.

With each song blasting out of our stereo I danced along celebrating life. I couldn't stop dancing in my seat. I was overflowing with gratitude for life. I was going to live again! After a few hours I was still moving to the music. I looked back at Ivy and she said, "Mom, you're scaring me. Dad, mom won't stop dancing and it's starting to freak me out."

"Me too" chimed Hannah.

I wasn't stopping. In between music we shared stories and we laughed and we bonded. I kept crying happy tears - Tears of thankfulness for a positive prognosis, for no more chemo, tears of thankfulness for John, for my beautiful daughters, for being able to go live again. This was what it was all about for me. It was about family and bonding and time spent together. Nothing else mattered to me. We all spent fourteen fantastic days laughing and living and healing - together as a family.

Holly Toner-Rose is Home Sweet Home!

Chapter Twenty-Nine

Wednesday, August 4th, 2009. Today was my first radiation appointment. Not knowing what to expect I asked John to drive me there. After we checked in, the nurses escorted me back to a changing room and informed me to wait there until I was called. John was told to wait in the waiting room. Soon a young technician called my name. She was young and pretty and as friendly as could be. All of the nurses throughout treatment had all been so nice. I was very thankful for them.

This particular nurse was very inquisitive asking me how chemo was, how losing my hair was, and could she see my baldhead, etc. I didn't mind the questions at all. In fact, I enjoyed sharing my experience with her. Then she told me how radiation would kill off any remaining cancerous cells. It was important that they administer the correct dosage to the exact same spot every time. To do this they needed to mark my body so that they could align me up perfectly day after day.

By marking my body they meant tattooing and so they did. I received my first two tattoos that day. They were just tiny pencil dots, one in the center of my chest and one on my side below my armpit. It was over before I knew it. So far so good. I had no complaints. I could do this. I dressed and found John with a smile.

> Holly Toner-Rose got her first two tattoos yesterday - just teeny tiny dots marking radiation. I asked for a rose but no luck. Ouch! Who does that by choice? I know I'm a bit wimpy when it comes to pain, but again. OUCH!
>
> Tammy likes this.
>
> Brian I think you should get a big-ass

302

butterfly tattooed on your hands, with John's initials underneath it.

Kate I didn't know butterflies had asses.

Brian It's a little-known fact. Most people don't know that they have breasts as well.

Kate I think you may be spending too much time in the sun

Everyone's humor on Facebook always cheered me up and I was able to forget my worries.

The next day when I returned I had my first exposure to radiation. Again, I was escorted back and asked to change. This time when the nurse called my name she led me in a different direction. We crossed a large room that had an enormous wall of equipment containing panel after panel of knobs and buttons and computers screens. Then we walked through a large 12-inch thick steel door. Immediately she asked me to lie on the table face up, with my arms up above my head. My breast was exposed as I lie on the table. Large mirrored panels surrounded me. The panels rotated around as she called out to her assistant, the corresponding digits to line me up. Moments later she slid a large angled mirror into one of the massive arms of the machine. She said they would be leaving the room during the radiation, but that they could see me on the monitors if there was a problem. I was told not to move - at all, and that I would feel nothing. It was not going to hurt.

I lay on the table as calm and as still as could be. My eyes were driven to the bright flashing red 'danger' light near the entrance. The large steel door closed and the red light turned to green. Once the green light came on, a sudden red beam with a constant low beeping noise bellowed out. It kind of sounded like a school fire drill or the noise you hear on the TV when they ring out "This is a test. This is only a test," but lower and constant. The red beam followed the ceiling, down the wall, to the arm of the foreign monster surrounding me and bounced off of the mirror plate facing me onto to my chest. I

303

closed my eyes and repeated "Just one. Just one. I can do this. Just one!" Eighteen seconds later and I was done. One treatment down, twenty-nine more to go.

That didn't hurt. I was okay. Although, I kept thinking back to what my friend Krys had said one night with her face all scrunched up and sympathetic tears in her eyes, "I hate to tell you this, but it's gonna hurt."

I thought to myself, "Was my skin going to slowly cook, day after day, from the intense invisible ray searing my delicate skin, until it shone with a slick crisp coating of a third degree burn? What the hell was going to happen? They doctors and nurses were telling me mild sunburn; was that the equivalent of what the chemo nurses told me - mild flu-like symptoms. Crap! They had lied! Are these people lying too? I have a sinking feeling I'm in for a world of pain."

And then I heard Dr. Zannis' words ringing in my head again, "One step at a time. Just take it one step at a time."

And so I did. I stepped out for my first training walk for the Susan G. Komen 3-day breast cancer walk with no worries about my pending radiation. I still had the illusion that I was in decent shape. I kept up with walking every other week during chemo so I assumed my body would jump right back into shape and I would be able to endure the sixty mile walk.

I met Katie at the mall for some indoor air-conditioned training. As we proceeded to do our laps around the mall, I could sense Katie was feeling impatient with my pace, so I tried to step it up a bit. I could feel my heart beating faster and faster, and my energy fading with each quickening step. We kept talking and I kept going. A few more laps and Katie asked me, "Can you pick up the pace some?"

Flurries of frustration raced through my mind. "Is she kidding? Hello? I just finished chemo and now I'm in radiation! Pick up the pace? Doesn't she realize that I'm pushing my body already? Do I really need to complain to every person so they get the fact that I'M TIRED? MY BODY

FEELS LIKE CRAP. I CAN'T DO EVERYTHING ANY LONGER. I DON'T EVEN HAVE THE ENERGY TO TRY!!!!!!!!! I FEEL LIKE CRAP!!!! GET IT PEOPLE!!!!"

Granted Katie didn't realize I felt bad. I didn't even realize I felt weak until I started walking. I was trying to shield everyone from my pain and keep it silent. I should have just been honest with people and let them know. No one can read my mind and I should not have been expecting people to.

She apologized nicely and so did I. She reminded me how great I was doing for our first training walk after months of chemo. She cheered me on as usual. We decided two miles was two miles closer to our twenty mile a day goal.

When I returned home I posted my progress on Facebook:

> Holly Toner-Rose had a rude awakening today. 20 miles for three days! Oh My Gosh! Laps around the mall for 1 hour about killed me today. I've got some training to do.

> Valerie You & me both, sister!!! I haven't done much walking in a week and today walked like 2 1/2 miles at lunch, dragging the entire way. We need to kick our butts into shape!!

> Holly Toner-Rose We can do it!!!!!!!

> Kate You were great yesterday! Okay, so we only did one mile. BUT, it was your FIRST training mile! And, while you are done with chemo, it's still not totally out of your body. I'm so impressed.
> PS - Metro was so NOT scary or dangerous. It seemed so much bigger when we were younger.

Friday, August 7th, 2009. I woke feeling anxious that

305

morning. I desperately wanted to go for a run. My body craved working out. Ever since I quit smoking exercise had become my source of antidepressant. During my college days I always worked out to keep weight off or to lose weight, but since I quit smoking I worked out to remain sane. Something weird happened when I quit smoking cigarettes. I'm not sure what nicotine did to my brain. Actually, I do know. The drug somehow kept me emotionally balanced. Maybe that is why I became addicted to cigarettes to begin with. Now I had to fight for my emotional stability everyday, so I ran.

Physically I thought I would be able to work out at this point, but I hadn't been ready emotionally. I wasn't ready to walk into the gym with a scarf on my head. I couldn't wear a wig to work out so I had no choice but to go bald (There was no chance in hell for that) or I could wear a scarf.

Why couldn't I just put the scarf on and walk out with my head held high? I didn't care what all of the people at the gym thought. I didn't know any of them so why was I so scared? I didn't want people to look at me. I didn't want them to look at me even when I did have hair. I still carried insecurities that people didn't like me, hair or no hair, so I didn't want anyone to notice me. Now I was more noticeable than ever. I also didn't want people to feel sorry for me. "Oh, look at that poor girl who has cancer." I didn't want to be a cancer patient.

I was bigger than this. I could do this. I cheered myself on for about an hour. "You can do this Holly. You can do this. It's not like people are going to point and laugh at you as you walk in the door. If anything people will be silently cheering you on. I can do this. I can do this. Damn it!"

I phoned Gretchen and I asked her if she could meet me. It was just the initial walk through the door. I just had to get through the door and I thought some emotional support would help. She happily said she'd meet me at the gym.

I stood in John's office with a scarf on my head repeating encouraging words to myself out loud. "I'm gonna do this. I can do this."

John responded, "I don't know why you even wear a scarf. You look beautiful without it. You don't even need it." I rolled my eyes in disbelief. I shook my hands up and down nervously and once more said, "I can do this," and walked out the door.

This was the first time I had walked outside of my house with a bandana on my head. I felt like the entire neighborhood was noticing my head as I drove by. Pulling into the parking lot my stomach sank and my breathing became constrained. "Oh crap! I can't do this! Where is Gretchen? Whew, there is her car! Crap! She's not in the car. She went inside. Damn it! What was she thinking? Didn't she realize when I said meet me at the gym that I was asking her to walk in with me????? I didn't need someone to stand by me the entire time I ran. I needed someone to get me through the damn door. Damn it! I can't do this. Damn it! Okay, it's just getting yourself through the door. You can do this Holly. No one is going to laugh at you. You can do this! You just have to do it once and the fear will be gone. Just this once. Just one! Just Do it!"

I took a deep breath, held my head high and walked. Biting my lips as I crossed the parking lot I searched for air. I searched for courage. I opened the door and proceeded to the counter. I tried to keep my head up and smile like I normally did, like nothing was different, like I did seven months ago. The attendant scanned my card and smiled back. Now I just had to make it across the floor and up the stairs. "I can do this. Just keep going Holly. You are almost there. You can do this! You can do this!" And I did. I made it to the top of the stairs and climbed onto the elliptical. "I did it." I felt a rush of relief sweep over me. I ran feeling life gushing through me. I was running again. I was living life again.

I returned to thinking about my meaning in life: to live and give. As I lay in bed each night my mind spun and spun trying to think of ways to give back. What could I do? What was I supposed to do? I knew I needed to give back, but how? I started to think about how cool it would be if I had tons of money to just give away. Then I realized I didn't really have much money to give away. It seemed that the recession hit us as well and we didn't have much left over. Here I wrote a book Live and Give and wanted to give back and now I didn't have any money to give. Maybe it was my time I was supposed to give back. Maybe I could go get a job and use that money to give away. Wouldn't it be great if my job was giving money away? That's it! I'll start a TV show, showcasing a different charity each week, and fundraise on the show and get sponsors and give, give, give! It would be like Extreme Homes but charities. It would educate the public on different charities and different fundraising ideas and draw people in with emotional stories. The Live and Give show. (I know - not sure what I was thinking - that I could do a TV show. Funny thing is I ran with it for a few weeks thinking it was possible. I tried to convince a bunch of friends to get in on it with me. A big no go. I've always been a bit of a dreamer.)

My next idea was to help out the breast cancer non-profit that was in the original Facebook posting from Shelley reminding me to perform a self-breast exam. I thought I could campaign here in Phoenix for them. I decided I was going to contact the founder to offer my time to help further her foundation. I loved the idea. (They asked not to be mentioned in my book incase you are wondering.)

I woke up in the morning excited to start spreading the word. I proudly slipped into my breast cancer awareness t-shirt they sent me and walked out my bedroom door to find my daughters there wide eyed and gasping, "MOM, you CAN'T wear that shirt!"

"What are you talking about girls?"

"Mom, please!" They desperately pleaded with me.

Deflated, I sulked back in my room and changed. Once in the car I asked them, "Do you girls care if I put a sticker on the car?"

"Yes!"

"Why would you be embarrassed by it? That is what saved my life." I explained to them the importance of their slogan and how it had reminded me to perform a self-breast exam and how it saved my life. I wanted to help do the same for other women. They still weren't buying it.

That night I lay thinking again, "What am I supposed to do then? I can't be a part of something that would embarrass my girls." I understood that to an eleven and twelve year old it could be embarrassing to have your mom wearing a slogan with a slang word for breast in it. I wanted them to be a part of it and be proud of me. I wanted them to be able to stand tall and say, "This is my mom and this is what she does." And then I realized I was supposed to start my own. The Live and Give Foundation. And we would emulate the other campaign but alter it to suit us. I knew the 40-something mother audience since that was me. I could reach out to them. That was what I was supposed to do: the Live and Give Foundation.

Katie and I went on one of our training walks and I asked her if she would be a part of it. Of course, she agreed. She then told me, "Yeah, the TV show thing, a little out of our league, but we can do this."

And so we brainstormed and at the end of our training walk we came up with, "Don't be a Chump! Check for a Lump!" We loved it. We would target all of the forty-somethings that believed their breasts were too lumpy to begin with to notice a difference or believed that they were too young to get breast cancer or it didn't run in their family so they didn't think they needed to worry. We were going to remind them on Facebook and the Internet and advertise in parenting magazines and billboards and women's expos. We were going to save lives just as someone else had saved mine. Katie was already a yes to be on the board. I decided to ask John, Gretchen and Shelley to be on the board with us. Each willingly said yes.

Summer was quickly breezing by. I had my port taken

out and made my daily trips to radiation. I was exercising. I was participating in life and finding my place again.

School resumed and I tried to resume my position as mother and nurturer. Over the past few months the girls began to turn to John. They went to him with questions, with homework, with hugs . . . he was the one they relied on. I was trying my best to find my place back into their lives without demanding it. I cried many a tear in my closet hoping to be an important figure in their life again.

At their back to school night we were informed the entire sixth grade class was going to Catalina Island off the coast of California for three days. The kids were going to be scuba diving, hiking, and exploring. The school was asking for chaperones for the trip. I desperately wanted to go along to be there with Hannah like I had always been. I picked up my application that night eager to fill it out, return it and start making plans.

My excitement was soon to be crushed. Hannah informed me that she didn't want me or her dad to go with her. It was part of her growing up and growing away from us. I boohooed over Hannah's request to Leslie and Janeen on one our walks. Leslie was applying to be a chaperone as well. Janeen went a few years earlier with her son. Janeen's advice was, "Go anyway. She may say she doesn't want you there but she will appreciate it." Janeen was the cool mom on her sons trips stocked with all the good candy and soda pop a twelve-year old boy could belly.

She told me how when she accompanied her kids on overnight trips she never saw her sons – she saw her son's friends though who would comment, "Your mom is so cool" and her son would be proud to have her there.

Janeen advised me to not give her that choice. She said in a bold tone, "I'm going Hannah. That is all there is to it." I loved her advice and promptly went home and exclaimed to Hannah that I was going to Cimi with her. She attempted a look of humiliation, but she made no case against it.

That evening as I sat filling out the application I completed the necessary information and then I had to answer questions as to why I was a good candidate to go and if there was anything holding me back from helping the kids in any way. I skipped the question and went to the next. I was going with my baby and that was that.

Tuesday, August 25th 2009. I worked out, went home and showered, got ready for the day, went to Target to buy back to school supplies for the girls, and then I was off to my radiation appointment. I was back. I was going about my day just like I had months before.

My last stop was Costco. I slowly pushed my cart around the stocked aisles. After the first half I realized that I was getting low on energy. I pushed even slower. I was having a hard time deciding what to buy. I no longer purchased red meat, anything with nitrates or any other trates for that matter, processed foods, high fructose corn syrup etc. My cart looked completely different than it did six months ago. It was stacked with fresh fruit and vegetables.

By the time I made it to the second half of the store my energy had depleted. Suddenly, I felt that I could no longer continue. It was the similar feeling of coming down with the flu, but worse. That feeling came upon me half way through Costco. I couldn't go on. I just couldn't go any further. "Damn it. I'm in Costco with a full cart. I can't do this. What the hell am I going to do? I just want to be better – Damn it! What do I do?" Tears started to roll down my cheeks. "Damn it! I can't finish this. I can't do this." Here I was crying in Costco again. I desperately searched for my phone and called John.

"John . . . I've done too much today and I can't go on. I'm tired. I'm just tired. I'm at Costco and my cart is full. I'm tired!"

"Holly, it's okay. You don't have to do everything. Just wait there. I'll come help you. I'll be right there." And he was. He was my night in shining armor. My love.

311

John rushed to meet me and pushed my cart down the aisles of Costco and piled them all into his truck. As I was driving home it struck me. I couldn't go to Catalina Island with Hannah. I wasn't better yet. Nor would I be in a month or two. What if I had one of my bad days? What if I had one of those days that doing a load of laundry exhausted me to the point of collapse? Granted, I would be done with radiation by that point, but not by much. And what about my hair? I still didn't have hair - just tiny fuzz. Hannah's friends had all seen my baldhead, but not the entire school. And kids would make fun of me. I didn't care about me, but I cared about Hannah. I didn't want kids to make fun of Hannah because her mother was bald. I couldn't do that to her.

I sat with Hannah that night and informed her that I couldn't go with her. I cried as I broke the news and explained the reasons why. The parents were going to support the kids and I may be the one needing support. That just wasn't fair to the entire sixth grade class or the other chaperones. My sweet little baby girl. She told me, "Its okay. Everyone has already seen you bald mom. I don't care if you'll be bald. My friends don't care if you're bald. Its okay mom." I loved my little girl so much at that moment. She really did want me to go. Janeen was right. She still needed me and wanted me around. I hope that never ever changes.

Chapter Thirty

Thursday, August 26th. I switched over to Dr. Quiet's new office to continue my radiation. So far my biggest complaint had been the long drive and the tiredness. I never did get the searing burns people had warned me about. Whew!

Sitting in the new waiting room in my dusty pink gown I read over a breast cancer pamphlet. I'm not sure why I picked it up. I wished I hadn't. I read about the possibilities of recurrence of breast cancer. It projected that women with large tumors and cancer that had spread to the lymph nodes had a greater risk for a reoccurrence. "That was me. Crap! Why did I read that?" I read further and it gave the statistic of women who had breast cancer and were still alive five years later. "How come everyone kept quoting five years? What happened after five years? Nothing I read in the past six months mentioned anything after five years? Why? Was it so bad that no one could write it down? Why? Did everyone die off? Why five years? I want to live longer than five years. I don't want to die young."

I was interrupted in my thoughts by Dr. Quiet's nurse calling me back. Dr. Quiet had a new regimen scheduled for me. She wanted me to do a seven-day power boost of radiation. She explained that they could give me a larger dose of radiation doing this using the mammography equipment. "Dr. Zannis said you were the best, so I trust you."

She led me to the back room. The room was painted in a golden hue. A massage table and mammogram machine filled the room. The nurse walked me up to the mammogram machine. The nurses and Dr. Quiet pressed and squeezed and pushed my breast until they were comfortable with where they had it positioned in the vice grip. They took a picture, took the film out and said we'll be right back.

I stood there with my boob clapped into the machine. I couldn't move. I could hear them around the corner struggling with the image. "No, we need to get her closer." They came back in and moved, squeezed, and tilted. Off they went once more with the film in hand. I heard the same pleas. "We need to get closer to the chest wall. B4, B6, A16" I heard steps once more. They all apologized and moved around me at a fast pace. They all new how uncomfortable this machine was. I told them all I was doing great and that I wasn't going anywhere. "Third time is the charm!" she said as she briskly left the room.

Third time was the charm. They entered again and hooked up two metal devices to the plates of the mammography machine. One on the top plate and one on the bottom. Next she hooked up a wire into each metal device. The long wire was connected to a robotic looking gadget. The gadget was a large white round cylinder container that looked like a trashcan, plastered with radioactive stickers. The nurse informed me that it would take thirteen minutes (Thirteen - not good).

They all left the room and I stood there alone with my breast imprisoned in this contraption. I was imprisoned. I glanced at the framed blood red poppies on the wall. Even the poppies looked sad. Flowers shouldn't look sad. "My head hurts. I want to move. Damn. Why five years? Five years is not enough. What happens after five years? I don't want to die young." Tears started to well up. I pulled at my gown and wiped my tears away. "Damn it. Don't cry. Just one! Just one. I'm okay. I'm okay. I'm not going to die." And then I was done.

The nurses came back smiling and laughed, "Please don't hate us. Are you okay?"

I answered with, "One down."

As I drove out of the parking lot tears welled up once more. I called John. I described the new procedure and how it hurt. I cried and I told him I didn't want to die young. He reassured me that I wasn't going to.

I spent the next few weeks feeling sorry for myself and many hours resting and Facebooking.

> Holly Toner-Rose Can someone please stop the world for a day so I can catch up?

> Holly Toner-Rose it sure is hard to cut out sugar. It's in my brownies, my ice cream and my movie milk duds. Impossible I tell you.

> Holly Toner-Rose is tired today. I'm calling it a personal day and I'm going to do NADA! ZIP! ZILCH! and I'm not going to feel one little bit guilty about it. (I can already hear my the guilt coming out in that sentence - Darn it! I'm going to have to work - or do I?)

> Holly Toner-Rose To the couch I go. ZZZZZZZZ!

> Holly Toner-Rose Damn! I'm tired again. I just won't have it. Sleepiness be gone. Be gone. Be. . .ZZZZZZZZZZ.

And then I spent an eye-opener of a day in radiation. I came home and posted this note.

> LIVE!!!

> Share

> Thursday, September 17, 2009 at 1:09pm

> September 16th. I showed up to radiation with a frown on my face and my eyes saturated with salty tears. Two months had gone by since I had finished chemo and my hair was a whopping half an inch. I looked like a boy. In my hopeful attempt

315

to look girly again I broke out my box of color me pretty hair dye. It did color my hair just not so pretty. Not only did I look like a boy, I looked like an ugly boy. I could have passed for Archie in the comic book, but worse. I spent the past two days crying. Again, crying over hair. Two days of life feeling sorry for myself. Here I was about to finish up radiation in a week with the prognosis that I was going to live to be 90 and I was crying over hair. Had I learned nothing the past 8 months?

As I sat in the waiting area feeling sorry for myself another woman walked into the waiting area. She was also dressed in the dusty pink gown waiting for her daily turn at radiation. Although, she was waiting with a smile. She was my age, forty, and a single mother with two children. She must have been so much more fearful than me through her experience having to go it alone. The worry she must have wondering what would happen to her children if her prognosis was not good. And then another woman entered with a smile. The second woman must have been eighty or so with the disposition of a cheerful twenty year old. Her home was an hour and a half away. Her husband had passed on and she was staying with her daughter while going through treatment - all with a smile. A third woman, also my age, proud to be a woman and proud to show her strength, opened up her gown to show me how her radiation was being administered. My radiation was an invisible beam. I couldn't see it, feel it, or touch it. Her radiation was injected into her. It was injected into her through thirty or so coffee stirrer like straws that the doctors had stuck into her breast one by one. Thirty or more of them sticking out of her breast! Again, she had a smile on her face.

I had to once more remind myself how lucky I was. I didn't have to go through the pain of someone sticking straws into my breast and then leave them there for a week. I didn't have to do chemo any longer. In one week I didn't have to do radiation any longer. I didn't have to lose my breasts. I didn't have to die. So, why was I sitting here feeling sorry for myself? Hair? So I chose not to feel sorry for myself. I chose to be happy.

So why am I sharing this with you now? Because I feel like I am one of lucky ones being reminded to live. I want to share that with everyone. I don't want you to have to go through cancer to learn this, just stop and appreciate your life! Live each moment, each day! Stop your work and your cleaning and go play with your kids. They are the treasures in this life. Stop and love your spouse. All the little things that may drive you crazy are just that - little. You fell in love and married so show your love. Stop looking for the bad. "If you are looking for the bad you will surely find it - Look for the good and you will find it too." So I'm asking everyone to do just that - myself included. Look for the good in your life, in people, in yourselves. Take a day and appreciate your life, your kids, your spouse, your friends and to all of you lovely women - your hair. Because even though I'm reminded it's not all that important in the big picture - it is one more thing you can be thankful for - even if it is a half inch long - it's hair, and I'm thankful for it and everything else I have!

Shelley I think I should start ever day reading this...Thanks!

Jerry This is awesome, Holly. Thanks.

Sheree I was having a really bad week and you made me feel better....love you Holly

Tammy Thank you Holly!!!!!!!!!! :) xox

Kim amen. and amen. so proud of your strength, holly!

Arin You are such an inspiration Holly! Thanks!

Jeremy Holly you are my hero and such in inspiration!!! Much love~Michelle

Emily Thanks Holly, I really needed to read that today...and I'll be reading it again tomorrow!

Vicki That is beautiful. Thank you.

Joanie This rocks!

John Rose I like your hair.

Holly Toner-RoseYou are all waaaaaay too nice. I wasn't looking for compliments but I Thank You! And I appreciate all of you!

Janeen I just read this, because I have

been too busy feeling sorry for myself this week.....Thanks so much for snapping me out of it...Love You!

Holly S.Thank you for this gift. You are such an amazing and beautiful woman.

Alisha Holly, I love you,sista, and so glad you are part of my life. You inspire me all the time.

Margaret Holly, what you wrote is beautiful. It made me cry and then I read Johns comment and it made me laugh...so simple and sweet and such a guy comment :)

Gretchen Holly, you are like a little angel!

Leslie Holly, you are an inspiration to all of us. A big part of that is your willingness to be REAL through this whole ordeal. You are allowing us all to learn how to handle this if happens to us, or anyone else around us. I only hope to handle any crisis in my life with an ounce of the grace that you have demonstrated. Thank you for your gift to all of us!

Marilyn Holly, we're thinking of you constantly!

Janice Holly, a couple of years ago I decided to surround myself with people who bring me up and help me to become a better person. This is advice that we give our kids on a daily basis. I am so glad that you and John and the girls are part of our lives. You make me a better person just through knowing you. I heart you and that never-ending smile of yours.

<u>Carol</u> You could never look like an ugly boy, Red. Wish, I had read this BEFORE I yelled at the kids. Hmmm.
XXOO

<u>Holly</u> With wonderful friends like all of you, I can get through anything!

Chapter Thirty-One

Sept. 23RD was my last day or radiation. I was done. Done with chemo. Done with radiation. Done with cancer.

Holly Toner-Rose It's official!!!!! I am a survivor!!!!!!!!!!!!!!!!!!!!!!!!!!!!!!!!!!!!!!!
Thank you everyone for all of your support the past 8 months. It has meant the world to me - every last thoughtful post!!!!!!!! Thank you!!!!!!!!!!!!!!!!!!!!

Jennifer , Ruth , Christopher and 10 others like this.

Frankie That's so great to hear!!!!

Kate Yeah!! Congratulations? We're going to party, on the party bus. Oh yea!

Kim and you did it with grace and courage and a lot of kick assness. go you!

Ernie Wonderful news!!!!!!

JeremyBGREAT NEW'S!!!!!!!!!!!!!!!!!!

Valerie Yay!!!!! So happy for you, and so proud of you, Holly! You are an inspiration.

Nicole Congratulations, you're an amazing woman!!!!

Arin Hooray Holly!!!! Congrats to you and your family! :)

Eric Way to go!!!!!!!!!!!!!!!!!

StacieYea! That's awesome news Holly! I knew you would kick it....you're a fighter!

ShereeYEAH...WOOHOO...SO PROUD

OF YOU HOLLY..SEE YOU SUNDAY AT THE LAKE:) LOVE YOU

Tammy YES YES AND YES!! :) XOXOX

Anna Holly has WON!!!!!!!

Hillary holly you rock!!!!!!!!!

Shelley Job well done, Holly.

My energy was starting to come back. I decided it was time to attempt a hike again. I had been looking at the mountain for months thinking, "If only I could hike again. Then it will all be back to normal." It was time. I put on my shoes and my iPod and headed out with my head held high. I came back home after one hill with my head down. "Not just yet."

Saturday, October 17th, 2009. I drove to Sedona for my a friend Krys' wedding. While I was at the reception my friend's mother came up to me and said, "You need to meet this woman. She had breast cancer last year.

After we had been introduced as breast cancer patients the other woman said to me, "It happened and I'm over it. It's not who I am." She didn't care to discuss it any further. I didn't mind. I was sick of talking about it myself. How was I? How was I feeling? Etc.

I understood her lack of enthusiasm on the subject. I also understood that every woman had to deal with it on her own terms. I had mine.

I questioned whether or not I should proceed with the Live and Give Foundation, recalling Dr. Zannis' words when I asked where help was needed. He advised me not to make it my life. After much consideration though, I couldn't help but conclude that this is my life. This is where life had taken me. Life took me here for a reason and maybe I processed it how I did for a reason and maybe I was Pollyanna about the whole damn thing for a reason and maybe this was one of my reasons for being here.

I took off my wig that night in the car on my drive home and I decided at that moment I was never going to put the wig on again. I was going to own who I was. All of me, teeny tiny fuzzies and all.

> Holly Toner-Rose Wigs be damned! I
> refuse to wear them any longer.

Wednesday, October 28th, 2009. This was my first appointment to see Dr. Ondreyco since chemotherapy. I made sure to bring John along with me - just in case. I didn't think there was anything bad at this point that she could tell me. Dr. Ondreyco did have blood tests done on me, so as a precaution and taking heed of my own words I asked John to accompany me. Dr. Ondreyco walked in with her usual smile on. She explained to me in detail about the Zoemeta injections I would be receiving every six months for the next three years. Initially, Zoemeta was given to bone cancer patients as a form of treatment and soon doctors discovered Zoemeta also reduced the risk of reoccurrence of breast cancer. Zoemeta was one more preventative drug I could take that upped my chances of survival a couple more percent. I was taking any percent I could get.

After Dr. Ondreyco left I dressed and John escorted me to the checkout station. I told him I would be fine for my Zoemeta injection. It was going to take an hour and there was no sense in him sticking around for it. We had no bad news and I had my laptop ready to write some more. I was fine. He kissed me goodbye and I waved him away with a sure smile.

Moments later the receptionist called me up. We scheduled my follow up appointment for January 28, 2010. That was perfect. That was one year from the day that John told me I had breast cancer. She couldn't give me bad news on the exact same day a year later. The chances of that were near impossible. I was given some other blood work and paperwork to pass on to the lab as well.

As I was finishing up Dr. Ondreyco returned clutching my four-inch folder of my paperwork. She informed me of the results of my lab work that she had forgotten to give me in the patient room. She said that my breast cancer blood work all came back clean. Then she said my CEA levels were slightly high and that she wanted me to have my blood work retested in six weeks. I asked her, "What are CEA levels?"

And she answered with, "Tumor markers." and walked away. I froze. I couldn't move. I couldn't speak.

I mind screamed out, "TUMOR MARKERS!!!! WHAT DO YOU MEAN TUMOR MARKERS? Oh My Gosh! Where is John? I sent John away. I sent him off with a kiss. Crap!!!!! I need John!!! Just one! Just one! JUST ONE!"

Dazed I walked into the chemo room. It was all happening again. I had to try to keep the tears back. "Damn it! I don't have my cell phone with me. I can't even call John. This can't be happening!!!!!!"

One of the nurses sadly sang out, "Aww, you're back."

"I'm just her for my Zeometa injection today." I told her.

My thoughts were screaming, "No way am I coming back to this hell. NO. NO!" I held back every tear that was fighting to come out. The nurse informed me they had a full house and I would have to wait in the reception checkout area until there was a seat. "Damn, cancer has a full house. It's everywhere."

Sitting back down in the waiting area I tried to push away my thoughts. "Slightly high CEA levels. . . Tumor markers. . . CRAP! THAT IS CANCER. THERE ARE MORE TUMORS INSIDE OF ME. JUST ONE! JUST ONE! JUST ONE! DAMN IT!" I picked up my notebook and tried to write hoping it would quell my worries for a moment or two. I couldn't focus on what I was writing much less the paper and pen I was holding.

Thank goodness a nurse tapped me on my shoulder and said, "We're ready for you, Holly."

I tried to force a smile and followed her. While I waited I quickly scanned the chemo room for a familiar face. No one looked familiar. I used to go on Fridays and this was a Wednesday. Were all the familiar faces done with chemo, or were they dead? I couldn't think about it any longer. As I looked about every person in the room was older once again. Not just older, I mean elderly, as in seventy-five to eighty-five. Could my luck really be that bad? Not only was I the one in two hundred and fifty to get breast cancer under the age of forty now I was going to be the one in thirty five that died from it. "Come on!!!! That just isn't fair!!!!!! Tumor Markers! Crap! I can't do this again! Just one! JUST ONE!"

Just one didn't work this time. Tears started to eek out. As I would wipe one away tear, two more tears took its place. Then I would wipe away two and four more followed. It was no use. My chin and lips began to quiver. I covered my face as best I could with my arm. Not wanting to cry in front of the whole chemo room. I had a hard enough time crying in front of people I knew. Did I really have to cry in front of these strangers? I didn't need everyone feeling sorry for me. I needed to be tumor free!

One of the nurses looked over at me and noticed my tears welling up. She rolled over to me in her chair and asked me if I was okay. I said, "Yes." - lie.

She told me, "Sometimes it is hard for patients to come back into the chemo room. You let your guard down after time has passed. Lots of patients experience this coming back. Is that what it is? Coming back to into the chemo room?"

I told her yes. She was right. It was hard coming back. It was that and so much more. I didn't want to be sick again.

The nurse Jan walked up with medicine in hand. I no longer had my port to connect to, so she poked and prodded for a good vein she could use. She found one and quickly hooked me up to my bag of Zoemeta. I pulled out my paper and pen and attempted to scribble away my worries. I kept having to stop writing to wipe away tears. Jan looked over at me at one point and said, "Is the I.V. hurting you?" If I spoke tears would flow, so I shook my head no. She asked again, "It looks like you're in pain. Is it burning?"

"No."

"It looks like you have tears in your eyes? Does it hurt?"

"No" I managed to get out in a whimper.

"I see tears though."

"It doesn't hurt. I just have tears."

"What's wrong?"

"If I talk about it I'm going to start crying and I don't want to cry," I said while crying. She gave me a comforting hug and left me alone.

The first nurse came back by and asked me if I heard bad news that day. There was no use trying not to cry any longer since the room echoed with my falling tears. I told her about my CEA levels and what Dr. Ondreyco said. She asked me if I smoked. I told her No (an old thought snuck in; wouldn't it be nice to have a cigarette right now to head off all of this danger for a moment or two). She said that smoking could raise CEA levels. With hope in my voice I asked, "Does anything else raise it?"

"No." She said reluctantly with a frown.

Inside I was screaming, "TUMOR MARKERS!!! I HAVE MORE TUMORS INSIDE OF ME. I DON'T WANT TO DIE OF CANCER! DAMN IT!! I DON'T WANT TO DIE SITTING IN SOME CHEMO CHAIR. I WANT TO LIVE. I'VE DONE EVERYTHING I COULD - DAMN IT!!! AND I SENT JOHN AWAY. I EVEN BROUGHT HIM WITH ME AND I SENT HIM AWAY. I CAN'T DO THIS

AGAIN!!!!!!!!!! "

Seconds felt like minutes and minutes felt like hours until I was finally finished. Another nurse came by to unhook me. She asked if I was okay. There was no use holding back now, so I explained it all again to her while crying. She immediately asked me, "Did you just finish up radiation?"

With a hint of glee in my eyes I sat up and responded, "Yes!"

"Oh honey, that is all it is. That happened to my neighbor too. Her levels were high and she even had a PET scan and it came back that she had two tumors. It was all just the radiation still in her body. It mimics tumors." I could have kissed her I was so happy.

I hugged her and cried out, "Really. So I don't have to panic for the next six weeks?"

"No. If doctor Ondreyco was worried about it, she would have had you redo the tests in a week. She said six weeks because she is waiting for the radiation to leave your body." I hugged her again and thanked her.

I wiped away my tears and walked as briskly as I could to my car. I opened the car door, jumped in, and started to bawl like a baby. I cried and cried harder than I had in months. "I CAN'T DO THIS AGAIN, GOD!!!! I CAN'T DO THIS. MY BODY IS NOT STRONG ENOUGH TO GO THROUGH THIS AGAIN. PLEASE GOD! DON'T LET THAT BE MY CALLING! I CAN'T DO IT. MY FAMILY CAN'T DO IT. WE HAVE BEEN THROUGH ALL WE CAN HANDLE. PLEASE GOD! I CAN'T DO IT AGAIN!!!!!!!!

I cried all the way home in fear. Later that evening I cried again to John and expressed how scared I was to have the possibility of it returning. "I don't ever want to get cancer again."

He looked at me puzzled and confidently said, "Holly, you don't have cancer anymore. It's not coming back." I prayed he was right. I prayed that night for me and my babies and John that we would not have to go through it all again. We just couldn't.

The next few weeks I pushed out any bad thoughts in my mind. I was moving on. I had the Susan G. Komen 3-day walk in a couple weeks and I had the Live and Give Foundation to focus on. We wanted our Check for a Lump website up and running before the walk.

The week before the walk I rushed around daily to accomplish my goals of completing the website and preparing/packing for the walk. After three days of typing, reading instructions, calling help centers, and throwing a few tantrums I completed our website. With my limited capabilities it turned out very primitive, but I was proud. I was proud to be a part of something good. We were going to make a difference. Maybe I had something more than a little light to give. Maybe my light was stronger than I thought. Or maybe all of our little lights together made us all shine brightly. I expressed these thoughts to Gretchen when she came by the house. She agreed. We were doing something good and should keep in going strong.

> HollyToner-Rose checkforalump.com is up and running. Yay!

> Holly Toner-Rose wants to thank John, Katie, Gretchen and Shelley. The LIVE AND GIVE Foundation would not have come to fruition without you. You all rock!!!! Thank you!

Friday November 12th, 2009. The Susan G. Komen 3-day race for the cure.

> Holly Toner-Rose OH MY GOSH!!! I have to wake up before 5:00 a.m. I should have trained for that part. I'm super excited to walk in the breast cancer 3-day. Yay!!!!!!!

The Susan G. Komen 3-Day for the Cure was one of the most rewarding experiences I have participated in my lifetime. I witnessed first hand humanity at its finest. Generosity, compassion, and camaraderie blossomed those three glorious days, like I have never seen before. The experience nourished my soul.

I returned home hopeful and filled with a natural high on life.

> Holly Toner-Rose I'm feeling a bit like a rock star after all of the cheering at the breast cancer 3 day. The experience was INCREDIBLE!!!!!!! Thank you everyone for walking with me. I love you all.

Thursday, November 19th, 2009 - I woke up and decided that today was the day. I was going to hike up to the top of the mountain once again. It had been a long ten months since I had been able to do this. This signified the end and the beginning for me.

> Holly Toner-Rose I have my iPod, hiking shoes and the mountain ahead of me. I'm making it to the top today!!!!

I didn't call Vicki or Katie or even John to go with me. I needed to do this by myself. I wanted to reflect upon my journey and savor each moment of my victory over cancer. I couldn't do this with others around.

I arrived at the base and I was ready to rock with my iPod in hand. Steadily I marched up the side of the mountain stepping to the beat. Higher and higher I climbed. I cheered myself on "I can do this!"

I recalled that day, ten months ago, while on that very trail, when I told my hiking buddy, Vicki, that I had found a lump the night before. I told her, "Surely it will be nothing." Clearly, I remember her saying, "You'll have to let me know how that goes."

Little did I know back then what was in store for me. I endured ten long months, packed full of treacherous moments and also beautiful moments. "I made it! I made it!" I told myself as tears flowed out into the open air.

As I climbed higher, I started to realize that my journey with cancer was much like the climb I was doing. The strong sturdy foundation of the mountain itself supported my every step just as my own foundation had supported me. The Saguaro cactus filled with strength stood tall and proud, withstanding any drought and every season, just as John did. A constant on the trail was the sunshine that brightened my day, smiling warmly and comforting me, just like my sweet Hannah and Ivy. The Palo Verde trees, like my friends, bloomed and filled the dusty mountainside with life. My family, just like the big boulders firmly planted on my sides were sprinkled with moss, only it wasn't moss that beautified them it was memories and seasons and time. Oncoming passerbys smiled at me cheering me on, just as my doctors had, knowing the hard trail ahead of me. And all of the small rocks on each side of the trail supporting it reminded me of all of those people I knew well and those I didn't know so well who supported me on Facebook. Ironically, I thought "What a beautiful experience this has been."

Reaching the top, I turned off my iPod, planted my feet at the edge of the rocks and looked around me. "I made it! I made it! I did it!" I thought to myself as tears streamed once again. I viewed the beautiful mountains scattered about the valley, each one erupting, right in the middle of a community. The valley below would have looked vacant without them. I reflected, "We all have mountains in our life. I believe they are all meant for climbing. Maybe we all need the mountains and their eruptions, to fully appreciate our lives and the people in them. The mountains added meaning to my life and I believe it added meaning to others as well."

My journey was over, I had learned to appreciate life a little more. I learned that John and our girls were the most important thing to me and that I wanted to fill our days with memories that would nourish our hearts and souls. I learned that I cherished my friends and my family. How lucky I was. I also learned that I wanted to give back to the community around me, and to those far off, hopefully making this world just a tiny bit better. I think that is all God really wants from us all to begin with. Maybe that is why He placed those mountains there in the first place - to remind us. Whether or not God choose to place another mountain before me was out of my hands. If He does, I will climb that one too. And some day, hopefully years and years away, I will climb the highest mountain to heaven.

I turned my iPod back on with Frank Black playing once more. "I DID IT! I BEAT CANCER!" Back down the mountain I headed. I was ready. I was Living and Giving.

AFTERTHOUGHTS

I can't say that I am happy to have had breast cancer, but I am grateful for the lessons I have learned, for the people in my life and the beauty in this world. My family is so much stronger having gone through this. I am stronger, John is stronger, our girls are stronger . . . our family is stronger. I am striving each day to Live and Give. I hope that you will do the same, whatever that may mean to you, and I hope that you remember to "Don't be a Chump! Check for a Lump!"

To honor my commitment to 'Live and Give', I pledge to divide any profits from the sale of this book accordingly. I will give fifty percent of any profits to our family income, to live a little more. My goal is to travel more with our children, experiencing this incredible world we live in, making more memories and creating stronger bonds that will last a lifetime. The other fifty-percent of profits will be divided among charities dear to me, including the original non-profit that reminded me to perform a self-breast check and saved my life. A percentage will also go to our non-profit, The Live and Give Foundation.

The Live and Give Foundation has started its first campaign, "Don't be a Chump! Check for a Lump!", dedicated to motivating women to perform self-breast exams, educating women about breast cancer issues and directly assisting those going through breast cancer treatment. Please join our campaign on our Facebook page "Don't be a Chump! Check for a Lump!" and sign on our guestbook on our website to receive a friendly monthly reminder to perform your self-breast exam at www.checkforalump.com.

Live and Give.

☺Holly Rose

Epilogue

Since I first published my book, I have been 'living and giving." I established the The Live and Give Foundation, Inc. aka Don't be a Chump! Check for a Lump! as a non-profit foundation, dedicated to educating and encouraging women and men to perform monthly breast self-exams and to have mammograms performed. We have sent out thousands of reminders to women and men through our Internet campaign. In October 2010, we formed a "Flash Mob" during National Breast Cancer Month, performing an impromptu dance before thousands of people and further spreading our message to "Don't Be A Chump! Check For A Lump!" As this book goes to reprint, we are preparing for our second Flash Mob event, to take place in October 2011.

I am very honored to say that in May 2011, we launched our "Wig Out" program, offering free custom wigs to breast cancer patients undergoing chemotherapy. To fund the program we held a gala event with art auctions, raffles, a dj and dancefloor with all guests wearing, you guessed it, wigs! We are forming relationships with many local doctors to refer patients to our Wig Out program, and have already helped several women purchase wigs.

Personally, I have traveled to Facebook headquarters to meet founder Mark Zuckerberg and share my story with his staff and to be part of MTV's "Diary of Facebook" program. I did finally make it to the Oprah show as an audience member during the very last week of taping!!! (Special thanks to my friend Cathy scoring us tickets!) Most importantly, I have been blessed with another year of this beautiful life and have spent the year with my girls and John making new memories to last us all a lifetime. I am Living and Giving! And I am, still, Cancer Free!!!!